Natural Support

For

Alzheimer's

Your Guide to using whole-health approaches for improving Alzheimer brain health and memory

Teri J. Dluznieski M.Ed.

Visit us @
RepairAlz.com

This book is dedicated to all my teachers... human and animal: and to the Earth. And to all the tireless caregivers- devoting time, energy, and heart to their work

ISBN 978-1508650454

For information on workshops and presentations contact:

Teri J. Dluznieski
Teri@zoogma.com
http://repairalz.com
Dluznieski, Teri J.

Index

Introduction

If you have been diagnosed with, or work with someone who suffers from Alzheimer's/ dementia or a cognitive impairment- you know it is a game-changer. While changes may be slow, and less noticeable because they do not happen all at once, changes are happening nonetheless. If you are reading this book, it is probably because you want to take a pro-active assertive course of action. You want to do the most you can, to minimise the damage that this is going to cause, to your life and the lives around you.

I mention this, because so often, when people are confronted with the idea or suggestion of making holistic changes to their life, they become very resistant. Sometimes they are intimidated, or overwhelmed. Maybe they don't know where to start. Or, perhaps they are just too comfortable with their unhealthy life-style to change anything. But in this case- things ARE going to change. They will either change around you/ them, or you can CHOOSE to make changes that can improve and deter the worst outcomes. Does it take some work? Absolutely! Is it worth it? That is going to be up to each individual to decide- how much and to what degree they want to incorporate a changed life-style. But the alternative does not leave a lot of room for doing nothing.

It is like an ancient proverb about Fate. We can sit still and wait for our Fate to come to us/ find us... or we can set out, and go forward to meet our Fate. Either way-- Fate is going to find us/connect with us/ happen.

This book is intended to support those who want to have a better functional understanding of the concepts around Alzheimer's, the brain, and holistic nutrition and dietary choices. It is not a medical book, nor is it intended to replace a doctor's (or holistic practitioner, naturopath, nutritionist etc)... professional input.

It is intended to support the caregiver, or Alzheimer patient in understanding the range of options and strategies that can maximise quality of life, maximise and regain cognitive function, and minimise the emotional and neurological stress that accompanies this reality.

Each chapter contains information, explanations, suggestions and worksheets and guides to support integrating this information and incorporating it into daily life.

I invite and encourage you to let this be the beginning of your journey and that you find the support mechanisms that can help make the shift into a holistic happier lifestyle that is rich and rewarding, for you or your Alzheimer family member or patient.

There are moments in our lives that stand as anchors. Moments: someone we love dies suddenly. A break-up or loss of job/ home, the diagnosis of a critical disease. Those critical moments define us. A point in Time. That "moment" is a place-holder in our lives. There is a "before" that moment, where life is mostly good and happy. Our lives have been moving forward along a Path we have been following- known, clear, safe.

And there is the "After," That Moment. A Moment that brings momentous change. We may not have any idea what Tomorrow will look like- literally or metaphorically (symbolically). That Path before us is no longer clear, certain or Safe. We may not even be able to see a Path in front of us.   We may stand Frozen, in that Moment. We may choose to stay frozen, or be unable to move from that Point, because the one thing we do know, with absolute conviction: whatever we thought was going to happen, what has worked for our entire lives... what worked "Yesterday," no longer applies.

The Rules have changed. The Landscape has altered. Hearing the diagnosis of Alzheimer's is one of those moments.

You may know someone who has gone through this: the

parent of a friend or colleague, a distant relative. You may have a vague and general awareness and understanding of the conditions.

Now it is you going through this. And suddenly you're feeling painfully uninformed. What you don't know or really fully understand becomes overwhelming and even terrifying.

You begin to read. You research online. You talk with your doctor. A picture begins to form: a sort of working definitions. Words like Amyloid Plaque and Tau protein, and connectivity become new words in your vocabulary. You are trying to wrap your head and understanding around the loss of vital essence, brain function and things that all of us take for granted every day.

Two of the most distressing words that enter into this vocabulary may be "progressive," and "degenerative." Those two words mean that Alzheimer's disease will continue to make more and more changes, and that those changes are causing the brain, and therefore identity and functions, to deteriorate. A death knell: a one directional journey that has no known cause, and worse, no known cure.

Now you begin to read about the stages and progression of the disease. If you are extremely determined, you may begin to study up on the latest findings and research. This is a valid and valiant undertaking: to become an informed advocate- either for yourself or someone you love. And you begin to read about different drugs (and side effects), new findings and new drug trials. The journey to understand and be able to impact change, can feel as hopeless and futile as the disease itself

Most of Mainstream Medicine, is outcome and cure- based: interventionary. This means it is excellent at intervening in the disease process and addressing symptoms. Quick fixes, such as broken bones, critical conditions and even in the treatment of some diseases and conditions. Doctors study for many years to understand how the body works. And what we know and continue to learn about the body, and the brain, is amazing. The more we learn, the better we can help. But in many ways, the more mainstream medicine learns about ways to "fix" problems, the more focused and narrow our approach becomes. This pill "cures" "that specific condition."

In this model, there is less appreciation, respect and

consideration for the bigger picture. Too often, our highly specialized medicine fails to look at cause and effect- that all too often, are not as simple as A causes B, any more than A cures B. The human body is a dynamic and complex family of many systems that work together and affect each other.

In terms of cause and effect, such as "smoking causes cancer," we know many people who smoke, who never develop cancer; and we know many people who develop lung or throat, cancers who never smoked.

We know that cause is a complex equation with many variables. Genetics, habits, environment, health, lifestyle, diet, exercise, etc. there is a very long list of probability factors. This is true with all disease, whether it is lung cancer or Alzheimer's.

With Alzheimer's the equation is even more complex. Diseases like cancer or fairly clear. HIV, cancer etc have actual organisms or pathogens that can be SEEN. A doctor can look under a microscope and visually see a causative factor- whether it is an actual pathogen, or something like a cancerous cell or tumour.

But with condition-type diseases, such as Alzheimer's,

there is no culprit. There is no Alzheimer's bacteria, virus or pathogen. Instead, doctors must look for evidence that accompanies the disease. There are criteria, when met, which indicate the likelihood that Alzheimer's is the underlying "cause."

Doctors will look for things like the presence of amyloid plaque in the brain. They can scan the brain to look for evidence of changes to the size and composition of the actual physical brain. They can look for the presence of amyloid plaque and Tau proteins. But, this is not the Disease.

We know these things are causing disruption in the brain's ability to function. We know the amyloid plaque builds up between brain cells, and that tau protein forms "tangles" inside the brain cells. This combination makes it very hard for brain cells to send information to each other, and that different areas of the brain struggle to communicate with each other. This demonstrates as the growing struggle to remember things, growing confusion and memory lapses.

But- what causes the plaques and tangles to form in the first place?? Are these things Causes, or are these things the result of something else in a longer chain of events?

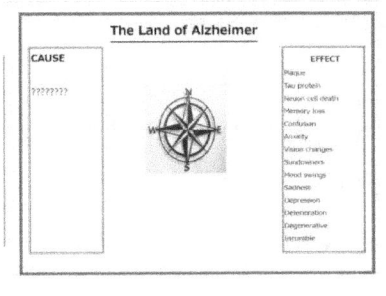

Imagine the Land of Alzheimer was a Map, with cause and effect as the compass. The Land to the East is well mapped and known. The symptoms, effects and outcomes are known with precise clarity. The precise timelines might be less precise, and extremes (?) might vary from one person to the next. But almost all medical doctors can look at test results and assess the level of progression (what stage of progression and deterioration). They can give fairly accurate predictions and estimates of what to expect, in what time frames. And they can also assess the ultimate Destination/ outcome. If this scenario was a door, or a road, it is a one-way route. A Dead End.

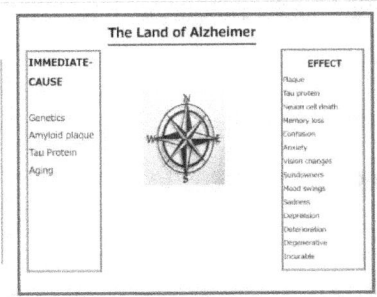

Now, the land to the West, is less known, less mapped. The land of causes. The land of "immediate causes" is a little better known. In this scenario, we move a few of the effects, like Amyloid Plaque and Tau proteins into a Causes column. These things CAUSE those other symptoms to happen. They are causes, as much as they are "disease." This region of immediate cause, is the land where genetics, Tau protein, amyloid plaques and aging are located (note, some of these things are both immediate cause, and immediate effect- living to both the left and right of the Middle.

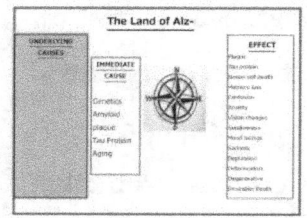

Unfortunately, on most Medical maps, this world is flat. The map/ world ends at the edge of "immediate causes." The area/ land further to the West is blank. This is the area/ Land of underlying causes and contributing factors. To many medical practitioners, this is a foreign land, dangerous and scary. To most, the map simply seems to stop at immediate causes. To travel further West would risk the same kind of danger faced in the days of old, where Christopher Columbus sailed bravely west- while all men aboard ship were also in constant terror of sailing off the edge into some terrible abyss or void.

This is where holistic and natural approaches to medicine and health excel. Ideally both approaches to health and disease should come together, for optimal outcomes. Both approaches have vital pieces of an important and complex puzzle that is in need of solving.

In order to maximize the potential for improving and reversing the damage caused by Alzheimer's, and improve brain function, we need to shift the focus areas on the Map.

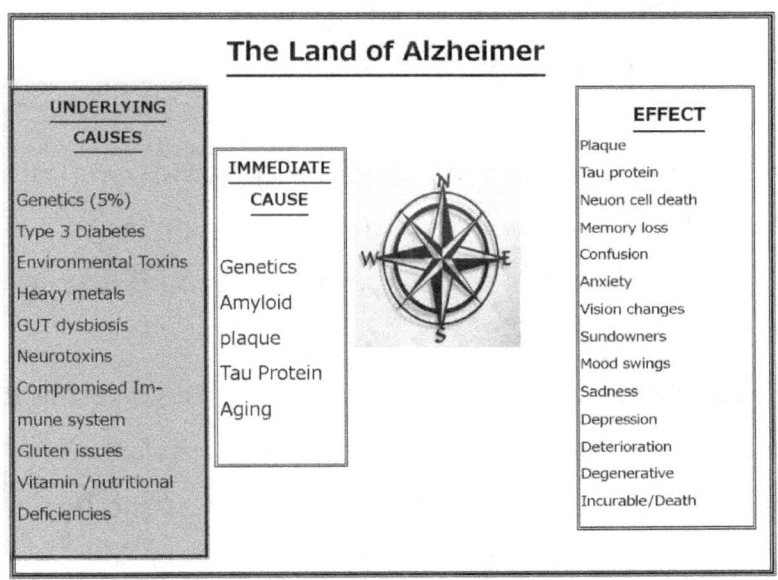

The Land of Alzheimer

UNDERLYING CAUSES

Genetics (5%)
Type 3 Diabetes
Environmental Toxins
Heavy metals
GUT dysbiosis
Neurotoxins
Compromised Immune system
Gluten issues
Vitamin /nutritional Deficiencies

IMMEDIATE CAUSE

Genetics
Amyloid plaque
Tau Protein
Aging

EFFECT

Plaque
Tau protein
Neuon cell death
Memory loss
Confusion
Anxiety
Vision changes
Sundowners
Mood swings
Sadness
Depression
Deterioration
Degenerative
Incurable/Death

Today, we tend to think of Alzheimer's as a disease. It has a clear set of symptoms (any many sub-categories with their unique symptoms), criteria and a predictable timeline of progression. It also has an equally predictable and assured outcome.

But what if we could expand the Map, and shift the focus of the map? What if we were to consider Alzheimer's as a symptom, instead of just as a disease?

In this scenario, Alzheimer's is a result of "something" as much as it is a cause of the symptoms we already understand and are trying to address. We need to explore that giant shadow area of contributing factors and underlying causes.

In this approach, we consider Alzheimer's as a symptom. From this, we work backwards. The question that follows... what caused these symptoms, or dysfunctions, to occur?

This is where natural and holistic approaches can step in and fill in the gaps. Natural medicine uses a "whole-health" approach and perspective to health and healing. It views and understands the body as an entire ecosystem (internal), and that it is also PART of an ecosystem (external).

In this way, the health of the brain and any deterioration is seen as part of the whole body. The health of the brain should be and is a reflection of the whole-body health. Think about this for a minute. The brain is THE most protected organ in the body. It is even encased in a healthy thick hard skull. All of the organs and systems in the body have evolved to assure that the brain gets optimal oxygen, nutrients, that assure its ability to move around in its environment, keep us safe and protected, and explore and learn. It also has mechanisms that maintain its optimal temperature, and remove all wastes (toxins and by-products) from the brain. There is even a special Blood-brain barrier, for added protection against foreign invaders. This ensures that bacteria, pathogens and germs cannot get into the brain. In fact, it can be hard to get medicines into the brain, because of this layer of protection!!

Scientists have even discovered that we yawn, to help cool the brain!! (cool science trivia). . Placing an ice pack (or bag of frozen vegetables) on the back of the neck reduced yawn rates between two study groups. This proved that yawning was temperature related, and not just boredom or fatigue. When we get tired, we don't breathe as well. This means blood is not being circulated to the brain as well and stays in the brain longer- heating up. Yawning forces more oxygen into the system, increasing heart rate (heart rate increases slightly on "inhale"). This sends fresh blood to the brain, which is also cooler in temperature, thereby lowering the temperature in the brain. Pretty amazing, eh?

So, we can begin to see just how amazing and dynamic the brain really is. Also, we can begin to see that it is also part of a system, the whole human body. The body is its support system that keeps the brain functioning and healthy.

When we consider the body and brain in this perspective, the next question makes more sense. What has happened in the rest of the body? What has caused these systems to stop doing their job? Why is the brain not getting or using its fuel (glucose)? Why is the brain no longer removing toxins?

What organs in the body are responsible for removing toxins? Are they so overloaded that toxins are now backing up, like a long line for the bathroom?

This is what we will explore in the rest of this book. We want to create an understanding of the "whole-health" approach to wellness, and specifically, the brain and Alzheimer's.

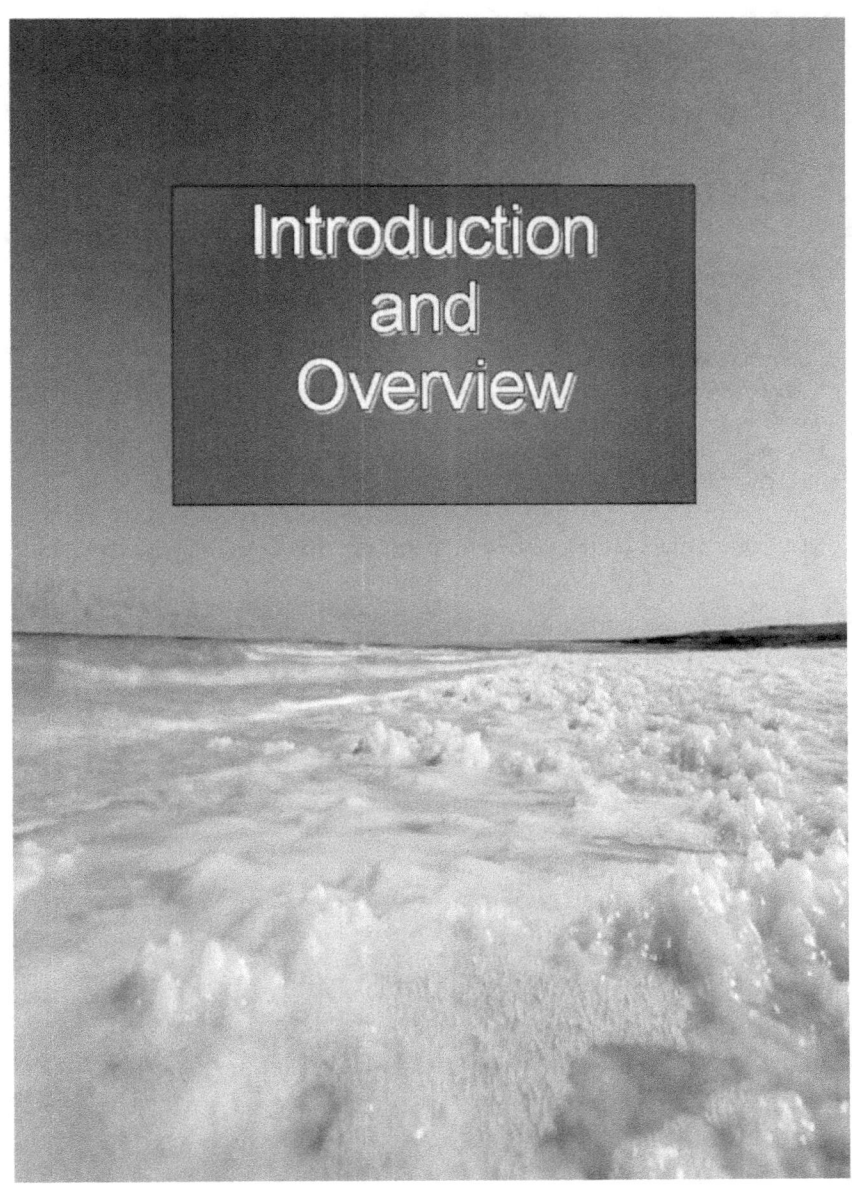

Introduction
and
Overview

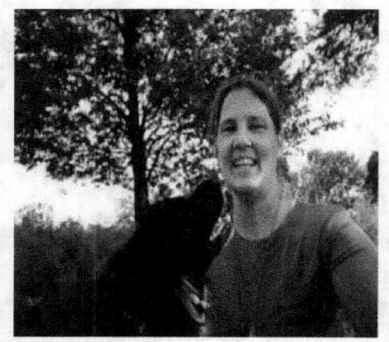 A quick and brief introduction. I am a holistic coach, with many years of traditional indigenous healing experience- which lends added perspectives, empathy and compassion to the holistic coaching I offer my clients. I am also a trained herbalist and bodyworker- because I understand that all the levels of health need to be addressed for your optimal health.

I have several books published as well as a large body of articles- many of which you can find on my website. You can read my full bio at the end of this book, and find out more about me by visiting my site, of finding me on my FACEBOOK PAGE

NOW, you picked up this ebook to learn something- so, on with the show!

Introduction and Overview

We will go into greater detail and description later in this chapter, but briefly- Alzheimer/dementia is a degenerative (it gets worse over time) disease where brain cells die off and changes in the brain affect memory, and the ability to learn new things. There are three basic stages: early, which usually begins as much as ten years BEFORE there are any clinical symptoms, the moderate stage, where most patients are first diagnosed.. when the beginning of symptoms become apparent, and the severe/ late stage, where the patient has lost the majority of basic functions and skills.

At a Glance- Statistics of Alzheimer/ dementia

- 5.2 million Americans suffer from this disease

- 6th leading cause of death

- 1 in 3 seniors suffers from Alzheimer's or a dementia

- 2013 cost US 203 BILLION dollars

Issues Specific for caregivers;

- More than 60% of Alzheimer's/dementia caregivers rate their emotional stress as high, or Very high.

- 30% of these caregivers report symptoms of depression

- Caregivers had 9.1 BILLION dollars in additional health care cost

What you will learn in this series?

- A medical and functional understanding of what takes place

- How dietary changes can minimise the uncontrolled activity and emotional outbursts/ frustrations

- Vitamins and supplements that support cognitive function and minimise stress/anxiety/activity

- The role and benefit of exercises and activities, and suggestions to implement them.

We will teach you how to improve:

- Day to day interactions

- Minimising stress of patient

- Maximising cognitive function

What is Alzheimer's?

There is no known underlying clear causative factor in Alzheimer's/dementia. Diseases such as HIV, Cancer or even the flu... have known, detectable pathogens. There IS a flu virus, which can be seen under a microscope: HIV and cancer, again... can be detected, tested, and visible proof, under a microscope.

Alzheimer's definitely exists. It would be so much easier to treat, if there were a clear causative agent. Some researchers are referring to it as "diabetes of the brain;" while other research is beginning to indicate that perhaps Lyme disease is an underlying pathogen-- that when it attacks the nervous system... one of the resulting possibilities is Alzheimer/ dementia.

There are a lot of theories. Still nothing definitive. Fortunately, modern research and techniques are learning more and more about the brain, about the nature of the disease/ condition itself.

According to some holistic practitioners/researchers, it is possible that HALF of the people with Alzheimer's may be misdiagnosed. They may, in fact, not have Alzheimer's, but be suffering from brain toxicity- due to a lifetime's exposure to toxins and heavy metals, nutritional deficiencies etc. Allopathic (mainstream) medicine seeks to find the magic bullet- both in terms of cause, and cure.

Holistic approaches understand that it is rarely "that simple." A wide range of factors contribute to a chronic condition. But underlying the holistic approach, is the understanding that removing interfering factors (toxins) and feeding the body with all the nutrients it can need and use-- are key to helping the body to help itself. Mainstream medicine wants to step in and give a quick-fix that does it FOR the body. Holistic medicine wants to help the body to help itself.

While mainstream medicine has yet to discover a cause or a cure, there are many treatments that are known to slow the progression of the disease. And both approaches can and often SHOULD be used in conjunction. Mainstream medicine does some things EXTREMELY well. Other things, less so. The real crucial element toward having any successful protocols for Alzheimer's (or any serious condition, and even just regular health-maintenance)... is to be informed, and understand and expect your practitioner to work WITH you and respect your wishes and questions.

If you have done your "homework," and your practitioner dismisses or downplays your questions and concerns... it is up to you to remember, YOU pay HIM/HER... not vice versa. It is their JOB to work WITH your wishes, NOT dismiss them or downplay their validity and possibility. Often, mainstream doctors are NOT that well informed about the latest alternative approaches. They dismiss information WITHOUT even really KNOWING anything about it. So, be prepared to be stonewalled by many medical doctors, who, at best, may acknowledge their lack of data. The best may be willing to investigate, or to monitor and support your protocols, offering what help they can, based on their knowledge. If not......

There is nothing written in stone that says you are married to this relationship. Shop around for a practitioner you like and whom respects your desires and at least shares a healthy respect, curiosity and interest in what YOU are bringing to this engagement. And if needed, create your own "team," of support- which might include a primary care physician, a nutritionist, a holistic practitioner/ naturopath, and herbalist. Acupuncture-- who knows. Each individual will find the combination of approaches that best serves their needs and preferences.

There are also many holistic modalities that can complement the mainstream medical approach and support. Holistic treatments are showing, in small scale (no big pharmaceutical money behind these research endeavours)... that it is possible to reclaim varying degrees of brain function and cognitive ability. Even mainstream medicine understands and agrees with the concept of neo-plasticity.

The ability of the brain to repair itself, and/or to have other areas of the brain to "learn" how to take over tasks for damaged brain sections. SO, if we KNOW the brain can repair itself, and that brain DAMAGE does not need to be "permanent," it becomes essential to take this information into account for the Alzheimer/dementia patient.

The goal of this book is to support the caregiver, family member, or practitioner in their goal of optimising brain function. In order to even BEGIN to address the possibility of restoring cognitive function, it is essential to understand the underlying mechanisms and contributing factors.

Before we can attempt to fix something, we have to understand how it works... and what is not working correctly. In other words, we need to understand what it is SUPPOSED to do. And we need to understand how it is "broken."

After we understand the way it should work, and how it is mis-working, we need to look at the contributing factors to the "breakdown." In regards to Alzheimer/dementia there are both "immediate" and underlying causative factors.

Let's look at the immediate causative factors first. But first, let's start with the "healthy brain."

The normal healthy brain

The brain uses up to 20 percent of all the energy/ calories used up by the human body.

The cerebral cortex alone (the most affected area in Alzheimer/dementia)- the front part of the brain where we process thought/ rational information... contains over 200 BILLION neurons and 125 TRILLION synapses.

A neuron is a nerve cell. Neurons are connected to each other. And communicate with each other. They are connected by thousands of **synapses**, to each other... neurons communicate through **AXONS.**.. like the pipe cleaners that connect tinker toys. So the pathway that information, or nerve impulses travel is: down the axon, to the cell body, to the synaptic terminus (the end of the pathway). An impulse will then trigger the release of neurotransitters that cross the synaptic cleft (space inbetween)... and then send the information down the line. (A very simplified explanation)

A neuron is like the HUB... the axon is like the long sticks that bind and hold them together. The difference between tinker toys and neurons.. is that they do not STAY locked together. And information has to cross the "gap" between neurons. Information, nerve impulses, flow down the axon, to a neuron-- where they "jump" across to another neuron-- via neuro- transmitters. **Neurotransmitters** are like chemical carriers... that "ferry" the nerve impulse across the "gap" between neurons from the sending neuron to the receiving neuron..... bridging the space inbetween. Something similar say to the pony express in history.

A carrier would bring a letter so far, where it would be transferred over to the next carrier. Passing the information along it's route, until it reached its destination.

Going back and forth, sending, receiving and retrieving information from the brain's complex and dynamic storage system.   If someone asks if you like chocolate. that question sends a "messenger" to where it knows information is 'stored," similar to a library with a catalog system (only we don't remotely understand the hows and whys of the way the brain stores information:)..

The brain has to "translate" the question, sort through the information for an answer, and send that "answer" information back through other areas of the brain, to the mouth.. so you can say " OMG YES! I Love chocolate." and the warm fuzzy areas of happy memories are also stimulated as well.   A lot goes on, even in simple questions and every day tasks.

In the Alzheimer/dementia patient... the synapses and neurons are affected.

In the Alzheimer brain... it appears that the brain is changing, long before there are clinical, noticeable symptoms and signs. Alzheimer's affects the older population more commonly. And there are age-related factors that contribute to this.

Certain areas of the brain atrophies a bit more with age (less use, combined with the aging process). There is added inflammation in the brain (the body's attempt to counter invasive/ intruding/toxins?).. and there is dysfunction in the brains mitochondria.

Mitochondria are the energy-factories, inside our cells. They convert energy into forms the cell can use. This is similar to the way our body converts food, into energy that the body and organs can use. Only mitochondria are doing this on the smallest microscopic levels- INSIDE each cell.

In the Alzheimer brain, the mitochondria somehow lose their "integrity"... and this leads to the loss of function. This means the cells in the brain are not being adequately "fed".. And important to note, studies found that the dysfunctional mitochondria were located at the synapses of neurons involved with memory.

Is the mitochondria the very first domino in a long line of dominoes? That's hard to say.

Another component of Alzheimer's is the build-up of **amyloid plaques** in the brain.

Anyone who has gone to the dentist understands the basic idea of **plaque**. It is a substance that builds up and interferes with normal function. In the brain of the Alzheimer patient, pieces of protein, called **beta-amyloids**... clump together. These proteins come from larger protein that is found in the fatty (protective) membrane surrounding the nerve cells/ neurons. Amyloid deposits are particles of oxidized protein that build up inside all non-dividing, cells, such as the brain and heart. Amyloid buildup slowly shuts down the ability of the cell to function properly and acts as an irritant.

The beta-amyloid has a sort of 'sticky' characteristic, and gradually builds up into plaques. As the plaques clump together, they can block the information that travels from cell to cell/ neuron to neuron. The plaques clog up the area around synapses, like a traffic jam at an intersection, and the normal flow of traffic... or information, is disrupted. The Plaque, may also be the cause of the inflammation- as the body-brain knows this is something that does not belong there, and it triggers an **immune response**.

Another major contributing aspect is something called **neurofibriliary tangles**. That's a mouthful! While the amyloid plaque is something that affects the cells from the outside, tangles, form INSIDE the neurons.

Tangles are composed of a protein called **Tau.** The tau protein is a part of cell structure, called **micro-tubules.** But in the Alzheimer brain it breaks down, and is not broken down and disposed of properly. Instead, they get twisted up and **tangle** together... interfering with the proper function of the cell on the inside.

So the proper function and communication of the brain cells/ neurons... is compromised from the inside AND the outside. Eventually, the neurons are so challenged that they cannot do their job. And when messages cannot be sent between neuron A to neuron B... repeatedly-- the connection between those two neurons is broken, and dies. Overall there becomes a **loss of connectivity** between brain cells.

So all the remaining neurons are a bit like islands.. with

fewer and fewer boats traveling between them, and they get cut off from the rest of the 'islands.' without proper food-nutrients, and lack of 'exercise' they wither up and die off. Just like people.

And as those connections die off... it becomes harder and harder for information to get through... the brain has to work that much harder, to find alternate routes between "source" and 'destination"

So this is a basic... overview of the brain and how Alzheimer affects the normal function of the brain. And we have a fundamental understanding of cause and affects of the damage that is taking place.

But from a holistic perspective, we try to look at broader and bigger pictures. In ideal circumstances an organism performs a function. Holistic medicine tries to understand what stopped working, and what interferes with its own ability to regulate its health and repair or heal itself.

In regards to Alzheimer's/ dementia, we may never know definitively, what the underlying single cause is. It may be that there is no ONE single underlying cause.

But we can begin to look at some things that we do KNOW and see as correlations.. for example... heavy metals may not CAUSE Alzheimer... heavy metals, like mercury aluminum and copper... BUT, there tends to be an OVER abundance or excess of these substances in Alzheimer/dementia patients.

So it is important to test and remove any contributing factors, by detoxing the body. It is also important to incorporate protocols that can remove the plaques and toxins from the brain... helping the brain to perform the house-cleaning that it can no longer manage on its own.

Additionally, there are specific vitamins that tend to be associated with the presence of Alzheimer's. Low vitamin

D for example seems much more common in Alzheimer than in the healthy brain/ patient.

We will go into more detail on these aspects in each of the chapters in this book...

We will also teach the importance of the healthy GUT, so that the body can get all the nutrients that the brain needs, and perform its functions optimally.

And we will look at supplements that support the brain's needs in detoxing, optimising nutrients, and maximising brain function. Some of the supplements can support relaxed states while promoting clarity. Other supplements reduce stress, while yet others can support the brains ability to repair itself and grow new nerve cells.

We will also look at the importance of exercise and activities. All FOUR components need to be in place, in order for the brain to have its best chance of being healthy and repairing itself.

1. Toxins need to be removed.

2. The GUT and organs need to be healthy and functioning.

3. The brain needs optimal nutrients to FEED its needs

4. The brain needs physical exercise that stimulates blood flow, and mental exercise that stimulates nerve health.

How many Americans suffer from Alzheimer/dementia?

_____

How might you define or perceive "holistic" medicine, alternative medicine, and approaches? Be honest.

_____

_____

_____

_____

My regular doctor is very open, or not open-minded at all? _____

A few possible alternatives to complement or replace this practitioner might be (anything from another doctor, a holistic MD, a Naturopath, Chiropractor, Acupuncturist, Herbalist, Nutritionist, Health Coach etc:

_____

_____

_____

_____

_____

_____

Write a brief definition of:

neuron _____

neurotransmitter

_____

amyloid plaque

_____

neurofibrilary tangles

_____

mitochondria _____

List the four essential components of a holistic Alzheimer's Protocol:

1._____

2._____

3._____

4._____

What habits or behaviours or issues are you trying to address or improve around an Alzheimer's/ dementia condition?

1._____

2._____

3._____

4._____

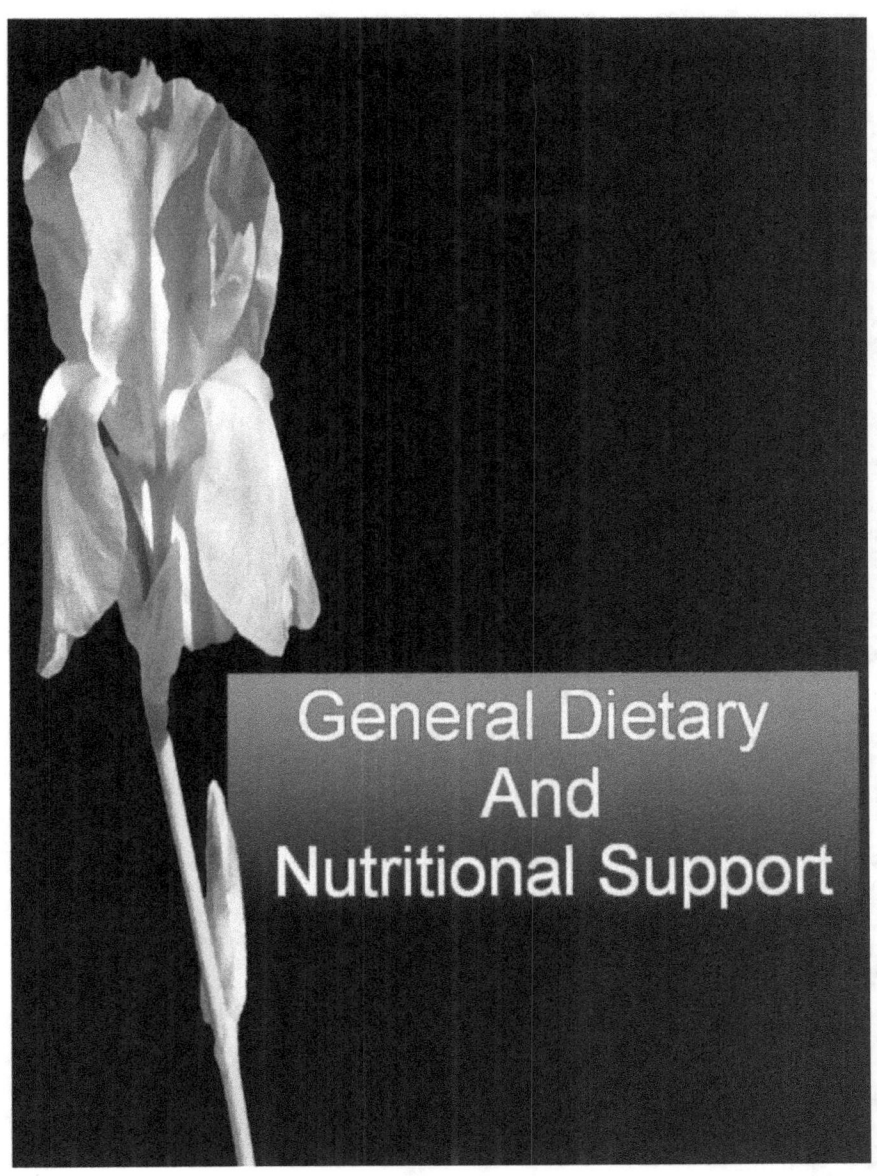

General Dietary
And
Nutritional Support

Diet and Nutritional Support

In this chapter we are going to look at a few different areas. First there is an overview. Then we will discuss general dietary and nutritional supports and why they may support the Alzheimer's patient. Then we will go on to talk about toxins and detoxing the body, with some easy to follow, and use suggestions that are generally safe and least-invasive/disruptive.

Overview

The importance and connection between the health of the GUT, and the health of the brain, and overall well-being.

First, I want to talk for a minute about the GUT. The GUT is so under-estimated in overall health and well-being. Digestion is where and how we break down foods and nutrients- determining what is needed from our food, and getting it where it needs to go, for the body to use.

The GUT also has the role of separating out the leftover waste, food, toxins etc.. and getting them out of the body.

The primary function of digestion is either through probiotic, healthy bacteria, and/ or via digestive enzymes (simplification, but enough to know, for our purposes). We will go into more detail on this, in the second half of this chapter, on detoxing. But for now, it is important to understand the importance of a healthy GUT.

The gut is a secondary nervous system, directly connected to the brain via the vagus nerve. We intuitively know and understand the role of the gut to our physical and emotional health. Gut feelings. Butterflies in the stomach. When the GUT is in distress, it is sending out signals of distress into the entire body, and brain. There are studies coming out now, that demonstrate connections between the gut, and depression and other emotional-mood disorders.

There are different bacteria found in the guts of autistic children, compared to "healthy" children; also between the guts of obese people, versus those with a healthy weight. The bacteria and health of the GUT is crucial for health, immune function, and well-being. We are what we eat, and we feel, based on what we eat. Food allergies can wreak havoc on physical, mental and emotional health. So how much of a role must this also play for the compromised brain?

It is important to understand the role of toxins, and the importance of removing them from the body. The liver and digestive tract, and kidneys are the body's primary tools for removing toxins from the body. This is why it is so important to support the body with whole and healthy foods and to have a good vitamin-supplement protocol.

The three types of toxins we are going to talk about are water soluble, fat soluble, and neuro-toxins

When most people talk about doing a detox, they are predominantly flushing out water based toxins, although any time the body fasts, it allows the body the chance to cleanse toxins of all sorts- this is because the body cannot divide too much of its energy in different directions. In a fasting state, for example, the body can then put its energy and attention in directions other than digestion.

This is an intrinsic component of fight-flight-freeze.
When the body is under stress, it does not do anything else, WELL. It is saving and conserving its resources for potential perceived need. Digesting lunch is not a biological priority when the body is worried about BECOMING lunch for something else. And while we no longer live in wild environments- those biological mechanisms function within the constraints of modern

culture.

This is why STRESS is such an important factor in wellness and well-being. When the body is under stress: and note, the body, like a circuit panel or power-strip, has a max-capacity for any-all stress. Stress is stress is stress... where it comes from, physical exertion, emotional stress, immune system, etc... the body has a limited/finite capacity to manage stress/stressors. And when it overloads, or goes beyond maximum capacity-- it begins to prioritise.

This is where we are more susceptible to disease, anxiety, even weight gain.. and, relevant to this topic-- we do not THINK or process as well. If you have ever been about to go into an interview, or audition... or a test, you can probably relate to high-stress and cognitive function. This is often what it must be like for the compromised brain... where it is struggling, in what is high-gear for its ability, to bring information into alignment. Maybe try to remember that when we have those moments of impatience in dealing with the compromised brain:)

SO, having touched on the role and importance of stress, and the idea that TOXINS are one important component of stress. They stress the physical body, trying to deal with both the presence and interference of the toxins... and the byproducts/waste that toxins produce..

This is why it is so important for whole foods that the body recognises. Everything you put in your body, or your patients body- the body has to process. NOTHING processes through the body without impact. So all the zero-calorie, zero fat fake substitutes... there is no free ride! And those free-ticket items... are even harder on the body, because they are so foreign, that the body is over-stressed trying to figure out what to do with them. Think of it like watching a foreign movie, without subtitles.

General Dietary Suggestions and Tips

Overview of Cooking culture and importance

The ideal diet will include lean meats and fish, fresh vegetables, and healthy fats such as olive oil, coconut oil, flax seed oil. In a perfect world, all food would be local and organic. I know that often we need to find realistic compromises. Organic meats and chicken can be very expensive.

There are some brands though, at least that advertise/promote themselves as never having been given antibiotics; note here that over HALF of all antibiotic use in the US, goes into our livestock. That's HUGE. And there is no way that cannot impact the health and nutrition of the animal, not to mention possible residues in the meat. You can also sometimes find in the larger markets, brands that are cage free, or free-range.

Find the closest to organic and free-range and/ or local, as you can work into your budget. Note- what I have found, and studies have found, is that it is possible to eat very healthy on the exact same budget- when all the junk-excesses are removed.

Making these kinds of changes can be difficult at first- but once you have made these shifts, shopping, cooking and meals are no more of a hassle than for any typical household.   And as more and more people are discovering their own health issues, gluten, colitis, or even heart disease and diabetes-- all of these necessitate dietary modifications.

So these modifications are not out of reach. Start slow, experiment, and find what works. It isn't easy, but the bottom line, is that if you are dealing with Alzheimer's.... that isn't going to be easy. But we can make it easier on everyone involved. It just takes a little practice and patience.

One of the biggest drawbacks to making the essential dietary changes, is that in our American culture- is that we no longer have a "sacred" element in regards to meals and mealtimes. It used to be that "be home in time for dinner," mattered. It was a domestic commandment, and people **stopped** at mealtimes. We sat down, we shared preparation chores (in some instances). And other things like television or phones, took a back seat.

This is no longer the normal practice in our culture. Meals are eaten on the run. Quick microwave meals and take-away have taken the place of Mealtimes. We live on the go. We are a "busy" society that is always in a hurry.

And I don't believe this is a byproduct or Modern Western culture. In Europe, there is still a social sacredness to meals and mealtime. So how have we gotten so far away from having regard for sustaining ourselves? Our diet, our food... is how we live, survive and maintain our health and lives.

So how do we find a balance? How do we not spend hours every day preparing specialised meals? If daily cooking is an issue, try cooking large dishes and dividing them into meal-portions that you can store in the refrigerator or freezer. A large pot of rice doesn't take much longer than a small one. And it can be stored in the refrigerator, and reheated quickly for a future meal. Or it can be later added to soup.

Crock pots are another handy and useful addition to the busy kitchen. Set it up, turn it on. You come back later to a cooked meal! I had a great time using mine, when I once determined it must be plugged in AND turned on... after waiting for many hours for soup that wasn't cooking

ANYway- back to our main topic.

Important terms to know and understand: **excito-toxin**, neuro-toxin. An excitotoxin is anything that over-stimulates, or excites the nervous system, nerve cells, system. Nerve cells ultimately are killed off through repeated over-stimulation. In simple terms, they are worn out and die. They die of exhaustion, sort of. There is an abundance of technical and medical information on this, if you are interested in specifics. Suffice it to say, the goal is to minimise excito-toxins. And in dietary terms, avoid things that may not be literal specific excito-toxins, but that over-stimulate the brain, nervous system and body.

Top of this list is caffeine. Sorry. This is one area that the Alzheimer compromise definitely demonstrates NOT ADD/ADHD. Replace with decaffeinated coffee or other non-caffeinated teas/beverages. Numerous caregivers have corroborated that the frustrated behaviours decreased when caffeinated beverages were removed from the diet. The brain is struggling for the neurons to line up and connect... being sped-up makes it that much harder.

Imagine you are learning a foreign language. If the person speaks slowly and clearly, you can follow and "figure it out." The faster they speak, the harder it becomes. The more words you "miss." Larger and larger comprehension gaps are created, until finally you, the listener, become utterly befuddled and confused. This is what it is like when the brain is being over-stimulated, for the compromised brain. I could make the argument that this is true for ANY brain, but let's just stick with the most relevant area.

One expert describes caffeine as, stopping the brains own inherent braking system. Caffeine binds to receptor sites, blocking normal processes, and so the brain CAN'T regulate itself to slow down, sleep, etc. Exactly what the challenged brain DOESN'T need! It NEEDS that extra space and time to do what the healthy brain accomplishes easily. Think of it like the learning disabled student.

They can get there, but they just need a few extra moments to connect the dots and put it together, than the "fast processor." Unfortunately, too many students become labeled as stupid, or "slow"... who are just as competent as their faster peers (although it might be interesting to study what dietary and nutritional impacts they may be struggling against;) the same is true of the challenged brain. Sometimes it just needs that extra time, with things slowed down, to make the connections.

Anyone who watches the frustration an Alzheimer patient expresses when too much is going on around them, should understand this phenomena. They literally can't think straight.

And note, as far as caffeine use goes- for anyone... that sluggish feeling in the morning, that "don't talk to me until I have had my coffee" mentality. That is drug withdrawal. Plain and simple. Your body has spent 8-12 hours detoxing and withdrawing from the previous day's caffeine.

If you, or whomever, has just had 7-9 hours or normal sleep, you should be waking up feeling refreshed and ready to go. The sluggishness, is detox and withdrawal, until the body has had it's "fix." If a heroin addict came down in the morning, and said don't talk to me until I've had my fix... chances are, they would be sent to rehab before they got across the room. Hhmmmm.....? :) something to think about:)

Decaffeinated coffee is not the end of the world. Honest! Neither are herb teas, and... water!

Sugars Culturally we are addicted to sugar. It is in almost everything. Sugar is instant food, instant-energy for the body. The body does not store sugar, it burns it. This is why we get the sugar-rush. It is why, intuitively, European cultures will mix a snack, say apples, with cheese; the fats in the cheese, slow down the metabolism of the sugar in the apple. Clever, huh?

Anyway, glucose, simple basic sugar, also speeds the aging of cells... can affect the aging of the brain, and studies have linked excess sugars and deficiency in memory, and brain health. OI! Also, there is a lot of evidence coming in that indicates that the Alzheimer brain has a sort of diabetes, and cannot, or does not burn glucose as its needed fuel. So, a high sugar diet, for an Alzheimer patient is similar to a diabetes patient. But the brain can burn some fats, very well, in the place of glucose. More on that later.

High fructose corn syrup: part sucrose and part fructose-- note that fructose is processed solely by the liver. The liver is crucial for many functions in the body. If it is compromised, it cannot do its job. Avoid high Fructose corn syrup in everything. But don't panic. Yes, fruits contain fructose, but they also contain higher fiber, intrinsic to the fruit, so while fructose doesn't tell the brain that its full, the fiber does. One of the many ill-effects of HFCS, is that it shuts down the brain/body's mechanism that says, "I'm full." A very likely contributing factor to the modern epidemic of obesity.

Avoid ALL Artificial sweeteners. Period. If something says it is sweet, but has no calories-- avoid it. The only beneficial no-calorie sweetener is stevia-based products-- and those are generally NOT being used by the food industry! Stevia is a natural sugar from a plant. It is not chemically altered or modified in any way. Your body recognises it and processes it- in fact, it has many health benefits.

Research shows that aspartame, under its many varied names, and saccharin, and sucralose all have negative impacts on mind and body.

Aspartame has long had connections to mood disorders, depression and brain impacts. I had my own personal experience in college, drinking as much as 2 liters/ day of diet soda-- having NO inclination that it could be harmful or have any affects. As the semester/ time progressed, I was feeling more and more overwhelmed, and struggled to cope. I was very near the edge of a meltdown (OK, probably in the midst of meltdown:).. when I came across a tiny article in the paper that talked about the connection between aspartame and manic depression/ depression. AHA! I IMMEDIATELY stopped drinking soda.

Within a few days, I began to feel like I had my life back. I could breathe, and function. It probably took a while for the chemicals to fully flush out of my body-- and I still had the normal stresses of college... BUT, I didn't feel like everything was out of control, or that I couldn't cope. I felt... sane:)

If you Google aspartame and the brain, you will find that NO amount of aspartame is safe, and it damages the brain. It leaves traces of methanol in the blood. Methanol= wood alcohol, NOT the good kind of alcohol! It converts into... formaldehyde! (embalming fluid). It is a neurotoxin, a carcinogen, AND it accumulates in the body over time. It destroys myelin tissue, the tissue, or protective sheath around nerve cells..the ones the Alzheimer patient needs to protect.

Additionally, the aspartic acid of aspartame, can cross the blood-brain barrier, where it attacks brain cells, as an excito-toxin, over-stimulating the cells and can cause... cell death!

EPA safe dose.. 7.8 mg. And yet our usage can exceed that as much as 250 mg/daily. And noting that the toxins accumulate over time!

sucralose-is made by using chlorine. IE bleach! Studies (which I personally do not trust) evidently show that in trace amounts it is not "bad for you" IE harmful. That's great (or not) for the healthy brain and body. But the Alzheimer brain and body is marginal, at best. So, even if this is accurate and true.... what might slip by without impact in an unchallenged system-- may severely impact the body-brain-system that doesn't have much or any latitude. Did that make sense? Some studies are showing a connection between consuming it, and aggression in small children...and since we are trying to minimise and eliminate ANYTHING that might be contributing to the stressful behaviours-- it's just better to find substitutes.

Better sweeteners: Honey, especially if it is local and raw. In fact, it has a lot of beneficial properties, and can even be used to help sleep.

Maple syrup, again, if local and/ or pure, real syrup, rather than most commercial store-bought brands that are made with artificial ingredients and "fillers."

Stevia, a natural plant that has many benefits for the body, no calories and is not an excito-toxin/stimulant. In fact, research indicates it has benefits for blood brain sugar levels, and is used in some instances for ADHD. There are now several commercial brands available. Ideally, try to get a pure liquid extract version, as it dissolves better than pure natural stevia powder does.

Even better, buy a stevia plant and use the leaves. Added benefit of living plants around and ready access to the sweetener:)

Also this cautionary information on artificial sweeteners, also applies to the artificial "fats."... and artificial colouring etc. Essentially, the closer it came from the Earth, the healthier it is:) If it is man-made and processed... avoid... is a good rule of thumb;)

Minimise pre-packaged foods, ideally eliminate altogether. Replace breads and pastas with whole grains, such as whole grain brown rice, quinoa (a grain that nutritionally is phenomenal. Ancient grain from Peru. Considered a super-food. Pronounced keen-wa) bulger wheat, oats, barley, etc. you can cook up a bunch in advance, and portion them out over the course of the week.

If you are using pastas, look for whole grain pastas, or pastas that contain various ingredients. My own preference is for one of the barilla brands, The box is yellow, and the ingredients list legumes, like lentils, peas, and vegetables... which, if I do need or want pasta... is an improvement over processed wheat grains, which may or may not be optimally healthy, because of potentially hidden wheat and gluten allergies:)

Again- remember, the less processed it comes, the better. The more of the work that needs to happen at the home-end... is a good indicator of healthier. Generally;)

I tried here to note some of the easier things to modify in daily diet. Foods that are readily accessible and affordable for the average budget. These are by no means the only food suggestions, or comprise ALL optimal modifications. Rather, let this serve as a baseline and starting point. You may find this shift in perspective and nutrition is adequate. You may find you want to take this to a higher level, as you see improvements and you want to increase the benefits:) Ideally, try working with a holistic practitioner or nutritionist. Then you can address specific individualized needs.

Lean meat choices And turkey is a good one to include, as it helps release tryptophan... the feel-good nap chemical:) note that to reach the brain, tryptophan needs to be paired up with carbohydrates:)

Sweet potatoes are another good minor switch. Ironically, they contain less sugar than white potatoes, and have a host of other potential health benefits, from helping to remove heavy metals from the body (toxins) and digestive tract, to helping reduce inflammation in brain tissue and nerve tissue, especially helpful here. The colour related phytonutrients may help with fibrin, which impacts the health of the myelin sheath in nerve cells.

The high vitamin and mineral content also makes them a good food for combating stress in the body. And remember, less stress equals easier management. They are naturally high in licopene, which improves mood and prevents the formation of inflammatory compounds.

Salmon is another great food to add to the diet. You just want to be very careful where it comes from, clean water etc- especially now that radioactive toxins are showing up in the pacific ocean. High in omega oils, esp DHA and EPA.. omega 3's which are crucial to brain health. They support brain health, and raise endorphins- the feel good molecules;) also, high in Vit D... where studies have found a connection between decreased D and depression.

Bananas. high levels of tryptophan, which is converted into serotonin -- the happy-mood brain neurotransmitter --strengthen the nervous system, and help with the production of white blood cells, all due to high levels of vitamin B-6 , prebiotic, stimulating the growth of friendly bacteria in the gut, tryptophan, helps to relieve Seasonal Affective Disorder (SAD)

Coconut oil- studies are showing huge benefits from raw fresh coconut oil. The essential fatty acids and the fact that the fat in coconut oil converts into lauric acid- which feeds the brain and nerves. Studies have shown cognitive improvement over time, taking approximately 3T serving/daily. Some studies are indicating cognitive improvement immediately after eating coconut oil. In which case, bedtime may or may not be the best time to have this. Coconut oil is a fatty acid that the brain CAN use for fuel, when it can't use glucose (sugar) properly.

There are a lot of easy ways to incorporate this into the daily diet. I use a "recipe" where I soften the coconut oil, put into a blender with a banana, an avocado, some other fresh fruit, sometimes some plain fresh yogurt, flaxseed etc... and turn it into a dessert snack. I then divide it up into single servings and store in the refrigerator. It stays good for well over a week, or longer. It has a thickness of pudding. You can experiment with the base recipe and find your own favourite.

You can also use coconut oil in place of butter or oil on potatoes, in soups or other places, making sure not to heat it too high and damage the nutrients. The information here is a little bit of info on coconut oil for brain/Alzheimer... but please, I invite you to Google this and read for yourself:)

Almonds- high in magnesium vit's E and B. magnesium helps relaxation. B helps energy. E helps muscle growth, Is an antioxidant that may protect brain cells

Lentils- -fighting folate, which helps make serotonin and dopamine, possibly explaining why up to half of people who suffer from depression have low folate levels

Grass-fed beef- if you DO want to include red meat in the diet, go with...Grass-fed beef contains more omega-3s and fewer omega 6s than its grain-fed counterpart, helping to mediate mood-wrecking inflammation in the body by increasing the energy available to the brain, creatine may help people better wrap their minds around problems.

Avocados high in fats particularly healthy fats. A good side addition to any meal or snack, if you are trying to add calories to maintain healthy weight. They are also anti-inflammatory, carotenoids support healthy heart, promotes healthy blood sugar regulation, which can smooth out those up and down cycles.

Tips and suggestions for cooking meals

Research has shown that the Mediterranean diet may lower the risk of developing Alzheimer's, and may even help prolong life in people with Alzheimer's. The Mediterranean diet has very little red meat. The diet focuses on fruits, vegetables, and nuts, with moderate amounts of dairy, fish, and poultry. Olive oil is an important source of healthy fats

A few other healthy alternatives and suggestions:

Whole oats, adding your own fruit, nuts or spices, is healthier and less expensive than buying pre-packaged portions with added sugars and other non-nutritive features. Oats and oatmeal, contain healthy carbohydrates and fiber needed to boost serotonin levels for up to three hours.

Eggs- you can make mini eggwiches using cupcake tins in the oven. Then you have a week's worth of pre-made breakfasts. You can add different toppings or seasonings to each, for variety.   Spices, herbs, cheeses, vegetables. Then you can just toast bread, English muffin etc, and have a quick ready-made breakfast.

Make something like a lasagna, make it with a lot of veggies, instead of as much cheese and dairy (especially if you suspect dairy allergies)... and cut into portions, and freeze/store.

Especially in summer, make a large salad that you can leave in the refrigerator- that way it is easier to make sure there are plenty of fresh options daily. I know if I have to MAKE the salad, I am less likely to EAT a salad; but if it is right there and ready to go... I will gladly choose that for or with my meal:)

These are just a few tips and suggestions. I am sure you can come up with far more than this on your own. And if you do have handy tips or ideas, please share them for others who may want the support.

Replace peanut butter with sunbutter, aka sunflower butter, or almond butter- both of which are very tasty and contain a lot of health benefits. It is extremely palatable, is NOT a goitrogen (depresses thyroid and body function), is high in magnesium as well as Vitamin E, as well as protein, zinc and iron.

Also.. Hidden food allergies, also known as 'brain allergies" can wreak havoc on health and emotional well-being.

A "brain allergy" is a food allergy that does not make you literally, physically ill. Nonetheless, some foods impact the body uniquely. Often there is no rhyme nor reason for the allergy, or the specific response. I have seen clinical footage of people being tested for allergies for the most common of foods: potatoes, bananas, grains, etc...as well as wheat and dairy, which are becoming more and more common.

The reactions to allergic foods can be anything in the spectrum of disturbance. Reactions can range from severe aggression, to giddiness, ADHD type symptoms, depression, anxiety or fatigue. Remember the sensitivity of the GUT... and the role of the immune system is HUGE within the GUT... so it... reacts...If you suspect there might be a food allergy, because you or your patient experience symptoms that are not "normal" ... it is a good idea to look into food allergies. You can try elimination of a suspected food. You should be able to tell within a few days. The tricky part comes if there is more than one allergen, in which case you might not feel better- because you are still being exposed to "something" the body doesn't like. Testing, or elimination are the two main ways to find out. Find a nutritionist, or holistic practitioner who has experience with food allergies/ brain allergies. Often you can find a chiropractor, who has studied "applied kinesiology" which is a way of "testing" the body for its reactions to different substances. The nice bit here is that medical insurance should cover these visits, and there is no blood-work etc... so the office visit/s cover the "testing."

What is your main first goal? Healthier nutritious food? Detoxing the body? Improving Mood and behaviour?

Do you find it easier to make changes all at once? Or slowly, a few at a time?

Make a list of FIVE foods that might be removed from the diet to help toward your goal:

1._____

2._____

3._____

4._____

5._____

Now, think of 1-2 substitutes for each of these foods.

1._____

2._____

3._____

4._____

5._____

How might you go about changing over to healthier choices?

_____

_____

_____

_____

_____

_____

_____

_____

Are these alternatives readily accessible? Do you need to go to, or find a different market?

_____

Do you shop at a health-food store or health-food section, for any of your shopping? If not, do you know where one is?

Look up and find the location of a health food store or co-op near you. Google, or yellow pages under health food, health, natural, etc... should help you find something in your area.

The local health food store or co-op in my area is
_____. It is near
_____ where I go to _____.
I could go there when I am going to

_____

If you have never been to the health food store, it can feel a little intimidating at first. Things don't look familiar, like the commercial grocery stores. But, the people are friendly and helpful. Ask someone for help. Tell them, "I have never been in a health food store of co-op. I am looking for a few items and was hoping you could help me find them." OR, "I have a few questions about _____ (a food, supplement or health related issue (not-medical)... Can you point me in the right direction?" Also, MOST health food stores and co-ops have a book section. Take a look at the books, on topics of healthy foods, vitamins, all kinds of interesting things. You can look things up in the books while you are there, if you prefer not to ask someone, right away.

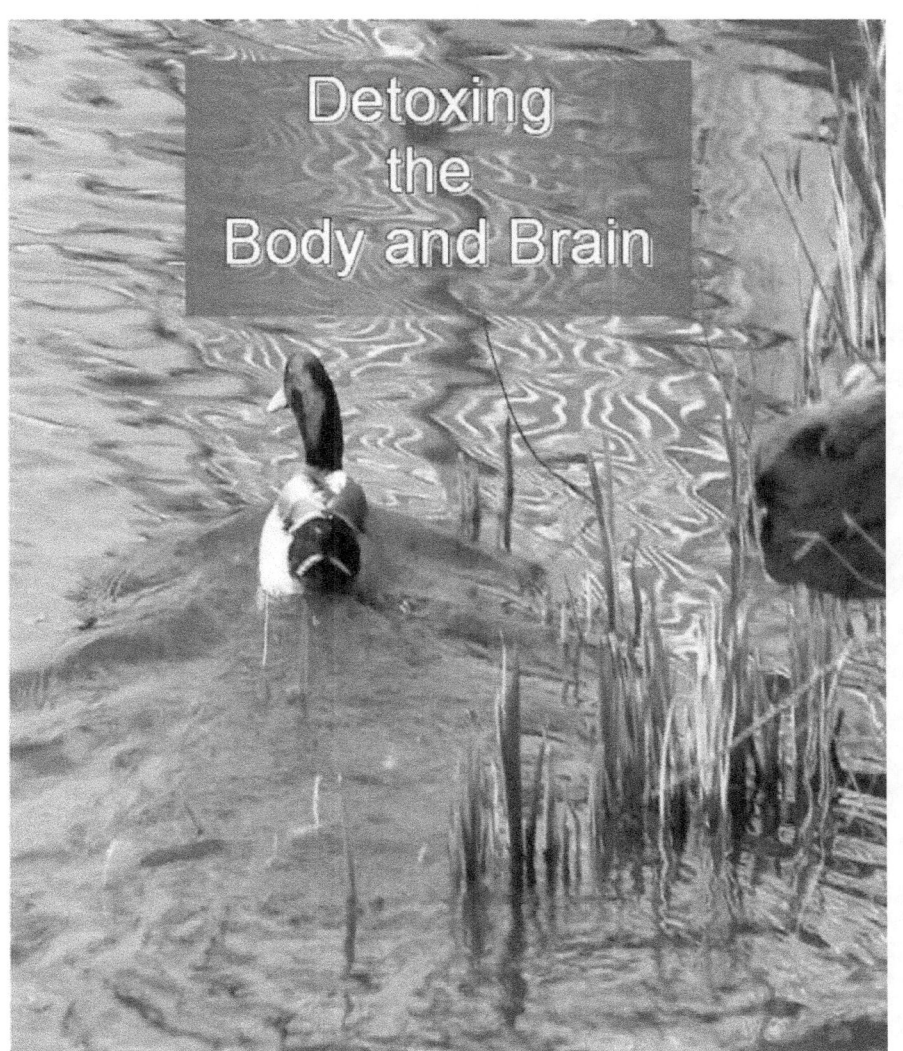

Detoxing
the
Body and Brain

Detoxing the GUT, Body and Brain

There are two important elements in a healthy gut and body. The first is eliminating toxins. The second is feeding the gut to replenish the healthy bacteria that it needs to function optimally. As noted in the previous section, there are two main components of digestion: enzymes, and (friendly) bacteria. Both of these are susceptible to toxins, which can interfere with their work, and even kill them And when the healthy-friendly bacteria dies, the bad bacteria (like yeast, for example), can become even more prevalent.

It is interesting to Note- over 500 species, and 3 POUNDS of bacteria live in your gut. Additionally, 75% of the immune system is in the GUT. The GUT is the enteric nervous system, directly connected to the brain via the vagus nerve. When it is in distress- it is sending out "distress" into the entire body, and into the brain-emotions. Sad or stressed GUT = sad stressed body, mind and emotions. Happy GUT= happier body. Also it is important to note- the body also creates a significant amount of neurotransmitters in the GUT.. so the brain NEEDS a healthy GUT!

There are things you can do to support the GUT to detox, especially if the GUT is compromised and needs help. It is important to maintain a healthy GUT and digestion for the above reason. Also, an unhealthy GUT can turn into "leaky GUT syndrome." Normally, the GUT is removing toxins and waste. In a "leaky gut," the GUT is so compromised that it cannot remove them. Instead, those toxins "leak" back into the body, causing inflammation and other toxin-related issues. Think of it like tiny holes in a garden hose... where water spouts out along the length of the hose. Only in this case.. it is the icky toxins, and it's leaking into your body!

- So- it is important to have a healthy GUT because

- GUT-emotion connection

- It creates neurotransmitters that the brain will need

- Toxic GUT can leech toxins back into the body

So now that we understand a bit more about WHY it is important to have a healthy GUT and digestion, let's look at some things you can do to make your GUT happy and healthy.

Detoxing the GUT

Let's start with a very quick overview:

The best way to detox the gut is to eat healthy foods.

Some things that can help support the removal of toxins from the body are:

Bulk fibers like **psyllium** can help to move foods through the digestive tract. And Remember to drink lots of water, to help flush things through.

Bentonite clay is a good detox support. It wraps toxins up safely and carries them out of the body. You can buy it from most health-food stores, co-ops, and even some of the larger food-chains that have health-food sections. You can also buy it online, from places like **vitacost**.com other vitamin suppliers, and even from Amazon.

Magnesium can help detox the gut, as a good dose of magnesium draws water into the GUT, helping the digestive tract to move things through.

Foods that help flush toxins through. Cabbage, onions, garlic, kale, spinach, whole grains such as brown rice and quinoa (keen-wa), sweet potatoes and squashes.

Avoid- pastas, breads, dairy, eggs, alcohol, and fried foods

Help HEAL the gut

On top of good healthy foods.. try eating small meals, so that your digestive system isn't overloaded. This way, your body isn't hit with more food, than it has ready-enzymes for processing.

Pre-biotic and pro-biotic: prebiotics fiber-based sugars, for example in from fruits and vegetables. These pre-biotics FEED the pro-biotics (good bacteria) so they are healthy and ready to do their jobs. And remember, any time you have antibiotics... add probiotics... antibiotics kill bacteria. ALL bacteria... they don't distinguish which is which... and so also kill off all the GOOD bacteria..

Additionally- you can add:

- L-glutamine, an amino acid supplement that supports healthy

- Marshmallow herb, and slippery elm – are both demulcent, they coat, soothe and heal inflammation.

- Colostrum is another natural GUT support. It is the first milk a mother produces. It kickstarts the GUT and immune system. In fact, babies who do not get colostrum within the first 24-48 hours, often do not grow healthy and strong. Many livestock do not even survive-- that's how vital and potent it is!! If you live near a dairy farm- you may get lucky- and be able to access fresh live-raw colostrum. If not, powdered colostrum is a good second option. Goat colostrum is probably the closest to human. And you can get goat colostrum in a powder form, either from a vitamin supply online, or from a goat supplier. I often get goat colostrum from Tractor supply company- which carries a lot of livestock/animal supplements.

- Add healthy fermented foods into the diet.

- Digestive enzymes-- and foods high in enzymes:

- fresh   greens

Detoxing the Blood and Urine

In order to detox the blood and urine, addressing kidneys is the key. The kidneys filter the blood, remove toxins and send them into the urine to be excreted safely. When the kidneys become toxic, or overloaded.. or create "stones," they cannot do their job of cleansing the blood and removing toxins, effectively.

Number one on the list of kidney supporting foods, is the **apple** (make sure its organic so it isn't sprayed with chemicals:)... Apples are high in pectin, which support many functions in the body, protects against cholesterol, and supports a healthy digestive tract.

Celery; is another. It is mildly diuretic and clears uric acid from the system. Is a traditional remedy for arthritis, gout and rheumatism. The plant is good, but celery seed is the more medicinal part of the plant.

Parsley very rich in minerals. Mildly diuretic. Helpful for many urinary problems as well as fluid retention. Minerals make it a good support for anemia.

Cinnamon is another great common household item that supports the kidneys and detoxing the body. It tones the kidneys and stimulates circulation.

Vitamin C- helps reduce histamine, which can cause inflammation, which can aggravate the kidneys. It is also a mild diuretic, so helps to flush out the body.

Nettle or "stinging nettle" is another excellent herb-plant-food for the body, especially the kidneys/blood. It is a circulatory stimulant, and a mild diuretic. It also removes uric acid from the system, relieving gout and arthritis. The leaves are extremely rich in minerals-making it an excellent remedy for anemia and "fatigue."

Red clover- is cleansing, mildly diuretic, and anti-inflammatory.

Burdock root- who would guess what a great plant burdock is... anyone with a dog in the country... is probably very familiar with this plant, or at least the burrs that get stuck in dogs, or horses fur/tails. Burdock cleanses the blood and supports the kidneys. It has mildly diuretic properties. It also breaks up uric acid, making it a good support for gout and arthritis. It is known to draw toxins out of joints.

Detoxing the liver.

There are two basic kinds of toxins: water soluble, and fat soluble. The best way to remove fat soluble toxins, is by supporting the liver, and the digestive tract. Additionally, hot saunas, and salt baths can also draw toxins out of the body.... through the skin! So can exercise-

sweating.   Plus, exercise helps all the body's systems function more efficiently...

But- there are things you can do, foods, and herbs etc that can support drawing toxins out of the body.

The liver performs more functions than we can imagine or appreciate. From removing damaged-dead red blood cells, to metabolising fats to removing toxins from the body.... In Chinese Medicine, the liver is considered "the general on the battlefield," overseeing a host of other functions in the body and coordinating many functions. This is why it is so important to have a healthy liver. It is a friend you want to keep on your side and, like your best team-player in a sport.. you want it in tip top shape and happy! :)

One of the very best things I have ever found for the Liver, is **Chaga.** It is a medicinal mushroom- hard woody, taking many years to grow on its host: birch trees.

It has a wide range of healing and medicinal components, especially regarded for its immune-boosting and immune modulating affects. It is most noted for its use in treating many cancers, hepatitis and HIV.

I have used it for years, as an immune-modulator, and adaptogen (as well as potent anti-oxidant).. against chronic non-responsive Lyme disease. Chaga contains many beneficial healing ingredients- polysaccharides, polyphenols, germanium and triterpenes.

Chaga is high in triterpenes, which are extremely helpful for detoxing the liver as well as combating high cholesterol. It is very high in beta-glucans- which are one of the components of its immune-modulating properties. Betulin and betulinic acid (derived from the birch tree itself, "digested" by the chaga to make it bio-available to people... are also powerful immune-boosting, particularly anti-cancer and anti-tumour..it even is used to heal ulcers...

Additionally it has a high ORAC, a scoring system for anti-oxidants... chaga ranges from 5,000 units to as high as 36,000 units to as high as 146,000 units-- given that it can vary based on geographical location.

And mushrooms in general, are considered a good way of removing heavy metal poisoning from the body as well as radioneuclides.

The good thing also is that there are no major contra-indications, OTHER than for those who have had transplants and/or are on immune suppressant medications.

Chaga is used in many forms. I think the best form of use, is as a tea- as the body processes "water" more efficiently than anything else, and the properties in the "tea" are very bio-available. Plus- it tastes great! Add a little cinnamon, honey, or other flavoured herb tea to it to make your own favourite blend!

Milk thistle is another great holistic-herbal way to detox the liver: it cleanses and supports liver function. It also helps detox the liver from toxins created by things such as alcohol. It also helps with regeneration of damaged liver tissue, and stimulates bile production, improving digestion. It can be taken as a tea or a tincture, and is readily available from health-food stores and some of the larger markets as a tea.

Chicory Root

Chicory also helps to cleanse the liver. It has been used in ancient traditions, from Roman, Persian and Indian medicinal traditions. It aids against jaundice, gallstones and liver stones, as well as urinary stones. It is known for supporting digestion/indigestion, depression and headaches.

Dandelion Root

Dandelion is a plant that is often under-appreciated. Especially by anyone who does lawn-care. But dandelions are great. From using their greens in salads, to using the root as a dye (magenta colour) It is rich in minerals, and supports many functions in the body. It is also good for detoxing the liver, and the blood. It stimulates bile and is used to help treat cirrhosis.

Organic Turmeric

Turmeric is experiencing a renaissance today. People are discovering just how great this herb-spice really is. It protects the liver and supports regeneration of the liver. It stimulates enzymes that help flush toxins out of the liver.

Peppermint

Peppermint is another under-appreciated herb. It is the

BEST first place to start for anything related to digestion or upsets. From gas, bloating, nausea, even projectile vomiting-the traditional remedy can work wonders. Just a few drops! But it also helps stimulate bile and helps to break down fats. It makes it easier for the liver to filter and flush toxins out of the body.

One of my all-time favourite detox supports is **cilantro pesto!** It tastes awesome. You can eat it in a lot of different ways- from a bagel spread, to mixing it into pasta.

Roughly- the recipe is: a bunch of cilantro, several cloves of fresh garlic, olive oil, Brazil nuts, pumpkin seeds, sunflower seeds, a little lemon/lime, and a touch of salt. Put it all in the food processor and mix until it becomes a tasty green paste! Store in the refrigerator- it keeps for a good week... if it lasts that long. And don't worry, those of you who don't care for the taste of cilantro... it isn't noticeable in the pesto, and it passes quickly!

Detoxing Brain-Based and Neuro-toxins.

By definition, a neurotoxin is any poison that acts on the nervous system. By nature, they are fat-loving and water-hating... which means they are in places in the body, which the most effective elimination, kidneys, lungs, or skin... cannot as readily access and remove. Often the body is saturated with fat-based toxins, and the fats become "neurotoxins" that deposit in the fatty tissue of the brain. This is why it is IMPERATIVE for Alzheimer and dementia patients to have a healthy GUT and liver!

Cilantro/Chlorella taken together. I also like **spirulina**, another **blue-green algae** for detoxing the body. Both chlorella and spirulina are what are called 'super-foods." And they provide a wealth of nutrients as well as healing and detoxing properties.

Apple pectin-- stock up on those organic apples!

High fiber green veggies- because they help to keep digestion working and allow the GUT to repair itself. It can't repair itself when it is still bombarded with toxins, and they are sitting, stagnant, in the GUT.

And then they can leak back and clog up the liver, and bind to fat-rich areas, like the liver and the brain. In this way, toxins are on a kind of repeating loop, circulating in the body, hopefully transported to the liver and intestines... but then leeching back into the body/system.

And it is important to note: **the brain is SIXTY percent.. FAT**. Dendrites, and synapses are about EIGHTY percent FAT. So it isn't hard to understand the importance of removing the fat-toxins/ neurotoxins from the body.

Putting healthy bacteria and enzymes back into the GUT

One of the biggest differences between traditional cultures and modern society, in terms of the health of their diets, is fermented foods. Traditional cultures, even modern French cuisine, is high in fats. But, all cultures have a tradition of fermented foods. The role of fermented foods, is to replenish the supply of beneficial bacteria into the GUT, which help to break down foods and digest nutrients, and eliminate waste.

There are many ways to include fermented foods in your diet. Many of which are easy to make right in the home. **Sauerkraut,** is nothing more than shredded cabbage, layered with salt, allowed to ferment for several days to several weeks. You can find recipes for making your own.

Yogurt is another form of fermented food. Ideally though, find a local organic brand, or better yet.... make your own. Again- very easy to do, and FAR more affordable than buying it in the market. Milk, heated to 160-180 degrees. Allow to cool to about 100 degrees. Add a small amount of yogurt to start. Place in a warm oven overnight (around 100 degrees) and in the morning you have a half gallon of fresh healthy yogurt! Look up recipes and instructions online. Or even better- get a book of recipes for making your own yogurts or fermented foods!

Kefir is similar to yogurt, but a "better" culture for its benefits to the body. You can get kefir "cultures" that turn milk into kefir overnight. You can also buy commercial kefirs now, as well.

Some other fermented foods- provided they are live, living, and not store-bought and nutrient-dead.. pickles, ketchup, relish.

Miso and Tempeh are also good sources, especially if you like Asian cooking.

Raw milk cheeses are another great source for fermented food healthy-bacteria!

A serving **1/4-1/2 cup of fermented vegetables/ day** is adequate to begin rebuilding and repairing the GUT. The added benefit, fermented food also help to draw out those nasty toxins! So a double benefit!

You can also take probiotics as a supplement. You can find these in most health-food stores, some of the larger commercial super markets, or online.

HIGH-enzyme foods to add to your diet

Papayas and pineapples are naturally high in digestive enzymes. These enzymes help to break down foods and nutrients. Do be careful to get NON-GMO and preferably organic fruits when possible. Especially papaya, as it is one of the TOP TEN GMO foods. Pineapple is high in bromelain, which breaks down proteins. Papaya is high in papain, which breaks the peptide bonds of those proteins, into amino acids.

Sprouted seeds, are another excellent source of enzymes. They are bursting with nutrients, literally, and contain up to 100 times more enzymes than other foods. And you can have fun sprouting your own seeds. It's very simple to do- and a cost effective way to add super-nutrients into your diet.

RAW nuts and seeds, are also naturally high in digestive enzymes. They are high in LIPASE- which breaks down fats, aka lipids..

And so are **raw fruits and vegetables**, they contain amylase, which breaks down carbohydrates.

And note- these are only some suggestions. This is not the total of information, just an introduction and overview. Enough to create understanding and awareness, as well as the beginning tools to create a healthier lifestyle. And as always, I actively encourage you to work with a holistic practitioner. A naturopath, a chiropractor whom may have an added area of nutrition, or a nutritionist, or qualified herbal practitioner.

Detoxing the Brain and Body: Guide and Worksheet

What are the two ways in which food is digested?

1._____

2._____

What organs help eliminate toxins from the body?

1_____

2_____

3._____

4._____

List three things that you can use to help remove toxins from the GUT

1._____

2._____

3._____

List three things you can use to detox the blood:

1._____

2._____

3._____

List three things you can use to detox Fat-soluble toxins

1._____

2._____

3._____

List something that you can use that detoxes the liver?
_____

List something you can use that detoxes the brain:
_____

Write down 3 different sources for adding enzymes to your diet-nutrition

1._____

2._____

3._____

The goal of this worksheet was to get you thinking about some of the easiest dietary changes you can begin to make to enhance the health of your body and improve the brain-health. Just by thinking about the questions, even if you had to peek, and look them up... you are using "data retrieval" mechanisms. In these kinds of exercises, more areas of the brain are activated and engaged.

So now, looking at this information, think of a plan that helps you begin to keep an ongoing active plan for implementing these changes.

The next time I go shopping I need to add these things to my list:

1._____

2._____

3._____

4._____

5._____

6._____

And note that this does not mean you will need to spend a lot more on your grocery budget, but rather some things will begin to replace others. Substitutions and alternatives, rather than additions-- in most cases.

One totally new food I might like to try is:
_____

I think the hardest part for me will be:

_____

_____

_____

_____

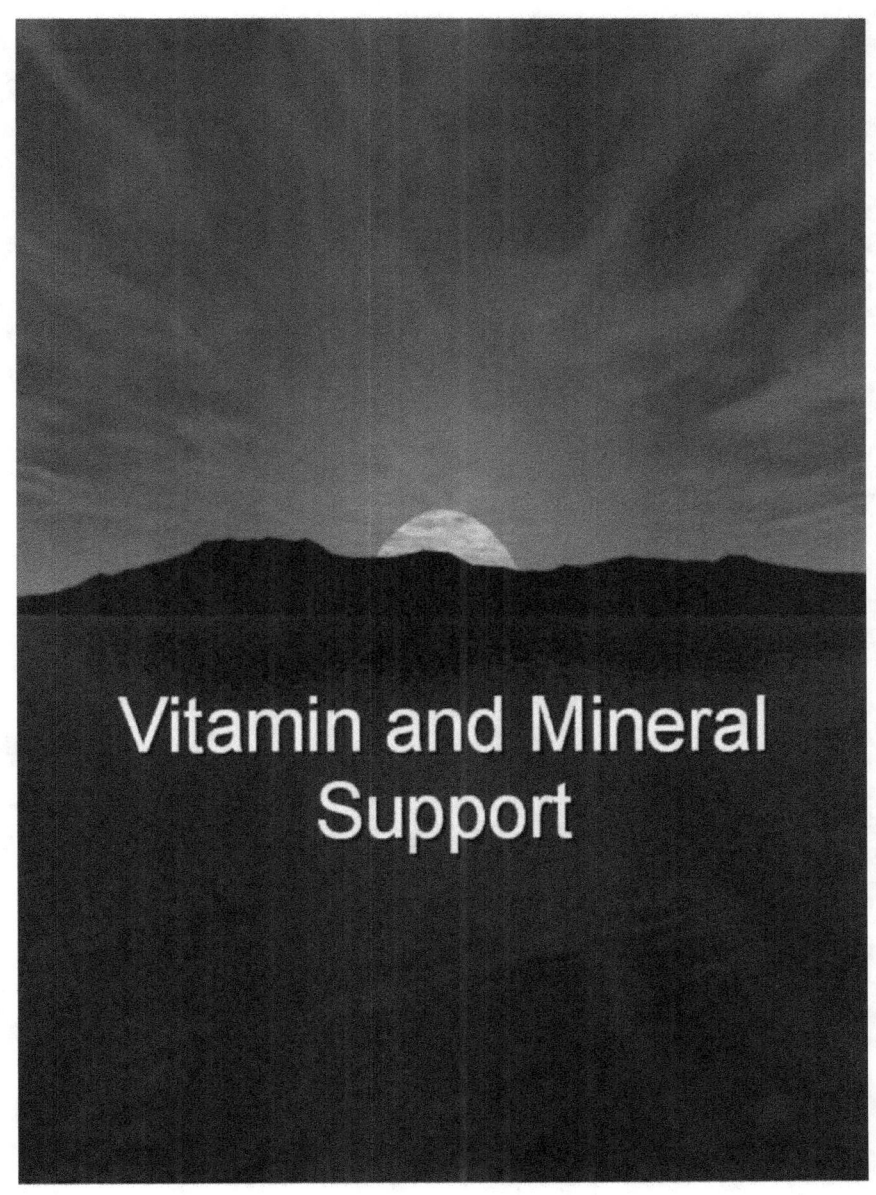

Vitamin and Mineral
Support

Vitamins, Minerals and Alzheimer's

We all know and have a basic ingrained understanding that Vitamins are important and vital for good health. We know that our foods contain vitamins, and that there are a variety of different vitamins. Each vitamin has its own specific function and role in supporting the body to maintain optimal health, wellness and functioning.

But most of us don't really know what vitamins are, and what they do, specifically, and WHY they are so important. They are so vital to health, that we are even told how much we need on a daily basis. We are also told how much vitamins are contained in given foods. They are even listed as what is known as the RDA.

RDA stands for Recommended Daily Allowance. But it is important to note that this long-standing standard of measurement is NOT a measurement of optimal requirement, nor does it account for situations when your body needs may exceed the recommendation. The RDA was developed to assure an individual could consume enough of vital vitamins and minerals etc... to stave off disease. For example- the RDA for Vitamin C was the level needed to NOT get scurvy... a disease that is caused by vitamin C deficiency. The level of Vitamin D, was based around the preventative dose to not get rickets. etc.

For example, I recently had whooping cough. When I googled holistic treatments for whooping cough, I came across information about Vitamin C. Apparently whooping cough consumes Vit. C, or... the body consumes and needs a considerably larger does of vitamin C than normal. This makes sense since vitamin C does support the immune system, and many other functions in the body. Many sites were referencing taking MASSIVE doses of Vitamin C, as high as "tolerance level" every 30 minutes for 24-48 hours to wipe out the pertussis.

I wasn't that brave or bold. I started with a lower dose of 500 milligrams every hour. I did not reach "tolerance level," (tolerance level indicates when the body begins to have light diarrhea). I slowly upped it, taking it more frequently throughout the day. I also had a sense that my body wanted-needed the Vit C, because I kept going back for more on a regular basis. The tablets themselves even started tasting good--- and I've never been keen on sour flavours!

I kept slowly upping my dose. Under normal circumstances, the body would not need anywhere near these levels. And, as the whooping cough did finally clear itself out of the body.. it stopped looking for Vit C. I reference this just to illustrate that doses for vitamins are based on.. normal considerations, and levels that stave off the most extreme of malnutrition based diseases. So our nutritional needs can vary according to our diets and our circumstances.

It is also important to note the distinction between **water-soluble and fat-soluble vitamins.** Vitamins A, D, E, and K are fat soluble. This means the body can and does STORE them in the body when you eat more than you need. It also means it is easier (not that easy) to "overdose" on a fat-soluble vitamin. Meaning, if you regularly consumed far in excess of your daily needs, the excess would continue to build up in the body's fats. Over time it could create problems in the body. This is not an overly common problem- especially in western culture which is so under-nutrient-fed.

The other vitamins, B, C in particular, are water-soluble. This means they reside in water. It also means any excess is NOT stored in the body, but is removed on a daily basis through the kidneys and urine. So, it is very difficult to overdose on the water-soluble vitamins, and... the repercussions of "overdosing" are less severe.

There are three sources for obtaining our vitamin requirements:

1. **Our foods**- what we eat

2. **Beverages**- what we drink, milk, juices etc.

3. **Our bodies** (the environment).. --some vitamins like K and some of the B vitamins can be produced by the bacteria in our body and intestines- another reason it is crucial to have a healthy functioning GUT that is not overloaded with toxins. Another example is Vitamin D, that is formed with the help of UV radiation, ie sunshine... on the skin.

In regards to Alzheimer's some vitamins may play a more vital role in supporting overall health, and brain health in particular.

Vitamin B:

The B vitamins play vital roles in cell metabolism. They are the energy vitamins. They are added to many of the popular commercial alert-energy drinks and formulas.

Vitamin B was once thought to be a single vitamin. Since then, research has shown that they are a kind of family of vitamins... 8 in total. They are distinct from each other- but are often found in the same foods. They are commonly referred to as the B complex. Vitamin B is the "energy vitamin." It supports the body's energy and can give a "boost" but without the nervous energy buzz that something like caffeine creates.

Each B vitamin does have its unique corresponding name/identity:

- B1 - thiamine
- B2- riboflavin
- B3 -niacin or niacinimide
- B5 -pantothenic acid
- B6- pyridoxine, pryidoxal, or pyridoxamine, or phridoxine hydrochloride
- B7 – biotin
- B9 Folic acid
- B12 cobalamins, cyanocobalamin in supplements

- the B vitamins play an important role in vital functions, such as healthy skin and hair,
- the mouth
- the liver
- they break down carbohydrates into glucose (energy)
- they break down fats and proteins, which supports the nervous system

A few specifics in regards to Alzheimer's

B6 or pyridoxine- supports the metabolism of amino acids, and lipids (fats). And plays an important role in creating glucose. It supports the synthesis of neurotransmitters, and hemoglobin (blood). It also helps produce niconitic acid (B3)

B12 — cobalamin: involved in the cells ability to metabolise carbohydrates, proteins and fats. It is essential for the production of new blood cells (bone marrow), as well as nerve sheaths.

FB9, Folic acid: is needed for normal cell division and aids in some of the processes for the production of red blood cells. It is also involved in some processes that support the metabolism of nucleic acids and amino acids (building blocks of proteins).

Vit B6 B12 and folic acid may play a role in slowing the progression of Alzheimer. A study showed a high dose B in an at-risk population showed shrinkage of whole-brain volume esp in areas known to be affected by Alzheimer. Study used 8 mg folic acid, 20 mg B6 and 5 mg b12

B 12 is usually best when taken in an injected form. Especially as it doesn't generally absorb well, particularly in the elderly population. Common deficiency symptoms list memory loss and cognition. This is especially true of the elderly, as the ability for absorption through the gut decreases with age. Another important reason to maintain a healthy GUT!

The preferred form of Vitamin B12 is methylcobalamin. Sublingual sprays absorb similarly to injections. These tend to be the more absorb-able forms of B12.

Another possible B vitamin that shows promise for treating and "reversing" the symptoms of Alzheimer's is **niacinimide** which **is a B3 vitamin.**

In one study it showed that taking this vitamin caused a 60 percent decrease in the Tau protein that causes the neurofibrilary tangles. Most studies indicate that it treats, but does not truly "cure," as the benefits are maintained only while taking the vitamin, and the benefits decrease after it is stopped.

Symptoms that may indicate niacinimide will be beneficial:

- Memory impaired; attention easily distracted; can't concentrate. Feels as if in a mental fog. Thought slowed. Difficulty comprehending. No longer reads as much as formerly.
- Unwarranted anxiety. Lacks initiative, not co-operative. Delays making decisions; evasive. Dodges responsibility; starts projects, never finishes.
- Frequently quarrelsome, mean, unreasonable, intolerant, opinionated, unhappy. Can't take a joke; little things annoy.

One anecdotal story indicated improvement on a general dose of 1,000 milligrams taken three times a day. And that spreading out the total amount was significantly more effective. Most people taking 1,000 milligrams daily, experience improvement within a few weeks. Some do show decided improvement more quickly. Apparently, it is also a treatment for arthritis, following the same protocols and doses. After 3-4 months symptoms had almost completely disappeared. So long as the patient continued taking the vitamin.

Note- as with any protocol, it is safer to start with a

smaller dose and build up. And, ideally-- to work with a holistic practitioner, nutritionist etc.

In one study, researchers gave mice the equivalent of a human dose of 2000 to 3000 milligrams of niacinamide, and the results were shocking. "Cognitively, they were cured,"..

It is certainly worth pursuing investigation regarding the potential success of the treatment. All treatments seem to have their base of "this cured my _____(fill in the blank). One of the benefits, at least, with vitamins.. in most instances, they will benefit the body, and do little to no harm if used knowledgeably.

Vitamin E:

Like Vitamin B, vitamin E is actually a group of 8 different fat soluble compounds. Tocopheral is the most biologically active form of Vit E. Vit E has many functions within the body, the most important being its role as an antioxidant. Specifically it is a fat-soluble antioxidant. It also supports enzyme activity and neurological functions. It incorporates into cell membranes, protecting the cell from oxidative stress. So it may be catching free radicals that can cause harm to brain cells, neurons etc.

It also plays a role in smooth muscle growth, and gene expression.

Deficiency can cause ataxia (lack of voluntary coordination of muscle movement/control...A dysfunction of the neurological function of the cerebellum that coordinates movement. IE poor balance and coordination)

Overdose can be associated with anti-coagulation.

And low vitamin E is associated with greater risk of Alzheimer's Studies showed that patients who took 2,000 units of vit E daily, were 30% less likely to die than the control group. And it appears to slow the progression from moderate to severe stages of the disease.

Vit D- is a fat soluble vitamin. It is also a group of compounds.

They are mostly responsible for the absorption of phosphorous and calcium in the intestines. In humans D3 is the most important form of the vitamin. In healthy people, it can be synthesized through the skins exposure to sunlight. Hence its nickname the sunshine vitamin. And the body has a built-in feedback mechanism so that the body cannot get an overdose of vitamin D through exposure to sunlight.

Vitamin D supports healthy bones and bone density. So it may be an important vitamin for those who are working to prevent osteoporosis.

Vit D deficiency causes rickets (a disease in children, characterised by soft weak bones that literally bend under weight. It can be categorised as bow legs).   Low levels of vitamin D are also associated with some cancers, and increased viral infections. Vitamin D deficiency is also linked to Multiple Sclerosis (MS).

Overdose can lead to hypercalcimia, may contribute to anorexia, weakness, insomnia and nervousness.

Vitamin D specific to Alzheimer/dementia

Studies link a connection between low levels of Vit D and death, as well as risk for Alzheimer, as well as poor outcomes on cognitive tests.   Research indicates that maintaining optimal levels of vitamin D may enhance the amount of important brain chemicals. It may also protect brain cells; and increase the effectiveness of **glial** cells (nerve cells), in nourishing damaged neurons back to health. Vitamin D may also help with inflammation, and immune boosting.

Additionally, Vitamin D3 and omega fatty acids may clear the brain of the amyloid plaques. (abnormal protein that clumps together forming sticky plaques in the brain) The study found that the active forms of D3 and omega oils improved the ability of macrophages (an immune system component. It works by wrapping up, or absorbing the foreign substance and removing it from the body/area) to absorb the amyloid plaques. It was also noticed that there was less cell-death that was usually associated with the amyloid beta plaque.

Minerals

Zinc is a micro-mineral. It is the 24th most common element on the planet. is an antioxidant, protects skin and muscles from accelerated aging. It also speeds up healing after an injury. It supports a healthy immune system. Zinc deficiency affects all parts of the immune system. It compromises white blood cell numbers and immune responses. Taking zinc can shorten the length of time it takes to get over colds.

Regulates genetic activity and balances carbohydrate metabolism and blood sugar.

A growing body of evidence indicates that zinc may preferentially kill prostate cancer cells.

Zinc deficiency can impair growth, including sexual growth.

A common sign of zinc deficiency is lack of taste. Inversely, a metallic taste in the mouth, can be an indicator of zinc toxicity (too much).

Zinc in relation to Alzheimer:

One of the components/ contributing aspects in Alzheimer's is that proteins lose their shape, due to damage. This leads to their clumping together. Zinc ions play a key role in helping proteins maintain their shape.

Magnesium

A key mineral in metabolism. It performs or supports over

300 chemical functions in the body. But the western diet generally fails to provide adequate supplies of this essential mineral. Magnesium is stored in bone, and deficiency can lead to bone loss.

It also supports energy production. Because of its role in energy production, low levels of magnesium IN the cells can be one factor that contributes to fatigue. It also plays a key role in regulating high blood pressure naturally. It also helps regulate blood glucose levels, in treating diabetes. It can also help in the treatment of migraines, insomnia and depression.

Magnesium and the brain:

In terms of support for treating Alzheimer, magnesium helps in the production of serotonin, which relaxes the nervous system and improves mood. Magnesium balances stress hormones, which can lead to poor sleep and insomnia. Magnesium helps with melatonin, which is needed for good and restful sleep.

Studies of Alzheimer's patients (mild to moderate) found those with low-ionized magnesium levels had the most impaired cognitive function compared to a control group

It plays a key role in regards to the activity of the NMDA receptor (brain cell receptor... where information goes in and out). Low levels of magnesium are linked to depression. Low magnesium levels have also been linked to inflammation (something else that needs to be controlled in the Alzheimer brain:).

There is preliminary research strongly suggesting a decrease in Alzheimer symptoms with increased levels of magnesium in the brain. Magnesium threonate, which can cross the blood-brain barrier.. may be an important part of pro-active treatments of Alzheimer's . magnesium-L-threonate (MgT), improves learning abilities, working memory, and short- and-long-term memory in rats. The magnesium also helped older rats perform better on a battery of learning tests. increased plasticity, or strength, among synapses and promoted the density of synapses in the hippocampus, a part of the brain that plays important roles in spatial navigation and long-term memory.

In general, the reading and information reading any connection between minerals and Alzheimer's/ dementia- - is more often the opposite of deficiency. The information indicates the problem in Alzheimer's is often the over-abundance of minerals in the body. Mercury and aluminum tending to be the highest. Also with copper, as an excess of the mineral causing problems in brain function. Iron and copper tend to be high, beyond normal levels in the brains of Alzheimer's patients, and can produce Alzheimer-like symptoms.

Copper, even at allowable levels, can break down the

barrier that keeps toxins from entering the brain. The accumulation of copper can also cause inflammation. It is found in many foods, and can even leech from copper pipes.

These minerals are also generally referred to as ' heavy metals." Testing for excess "heavy metals," is more common and accessible now. It can be tested through a hair analysis, or through blood-work

This is some of the reason why it is so crucial to support the body's ability to detoxify itself, and to support the removal of toxins and heavy metals from the body. This is especially true for the Alzheimer's brain.

We go into this in more detail in the detox the body chapter, but briefly.. a few ways to remove heavy metals safely from the body:

Bentonite clay: a teaspoon to a tablespoon daily, wraps up toxins and draws them safely out of the body.

Whenever possible, food-based approaches are always the best, and usually the safest ways to help feed and detox the body.

Cilantro is one of THE best detoxing agents, especially for heavy metals. A quick recipe for **cilantro pesto**, which contains a whole list of foods that detox the body:

- a bunch of cilantro
- extra virgin olive oil
- fresh garlic- 3-5 cloves
- handful of sunflower seeds
- handful of pumpkin seeds
- handful of Brazil nuts
- a little bit of lemon juice or lime juice
- a touch of sea salt as flavour

Put it all into a Cuisinart/ blender and puree. It should blend down into a nice paste. Use about 1 tablespoon daily. It is far more tasty than cilantro-haters might think. After eating it once or twice, even the most strongly opposed to cilantro find themselves enjoying it. Put it on bagel or toast, add it to pasta (do not cook it, add it in after pasta is cooked... so it warms up, but does not damage the nutrients). You may find a lot of ways to use the pesto, and it is doing great things for the body!

Vitamins and Minerals Worksheets

Which vitamins are water soluble and which ones are fat soluble:

A _____

B complex _____

C _____

D complex _____

E _____

K _____

Which vitamin is the energy-vitamin? ____

Which vitamin/s help the immune system? _____

Which one most helps the brain/ neurological function?

_____

Which minerals are often in excess amounts in the Alzheimer's Patient?

_____

List three ways you might incorporate into a regular diet, which will help remove heavy metals and/ or neuro-toxins.

1._____

2._____

3._____

My plan is to start by adding these changes to my diet:_____
_____
_____
_____

The next time I go shopping, I need to add these things to my list, or buy online:

1._____

2._____

3._____

4._____

5._____

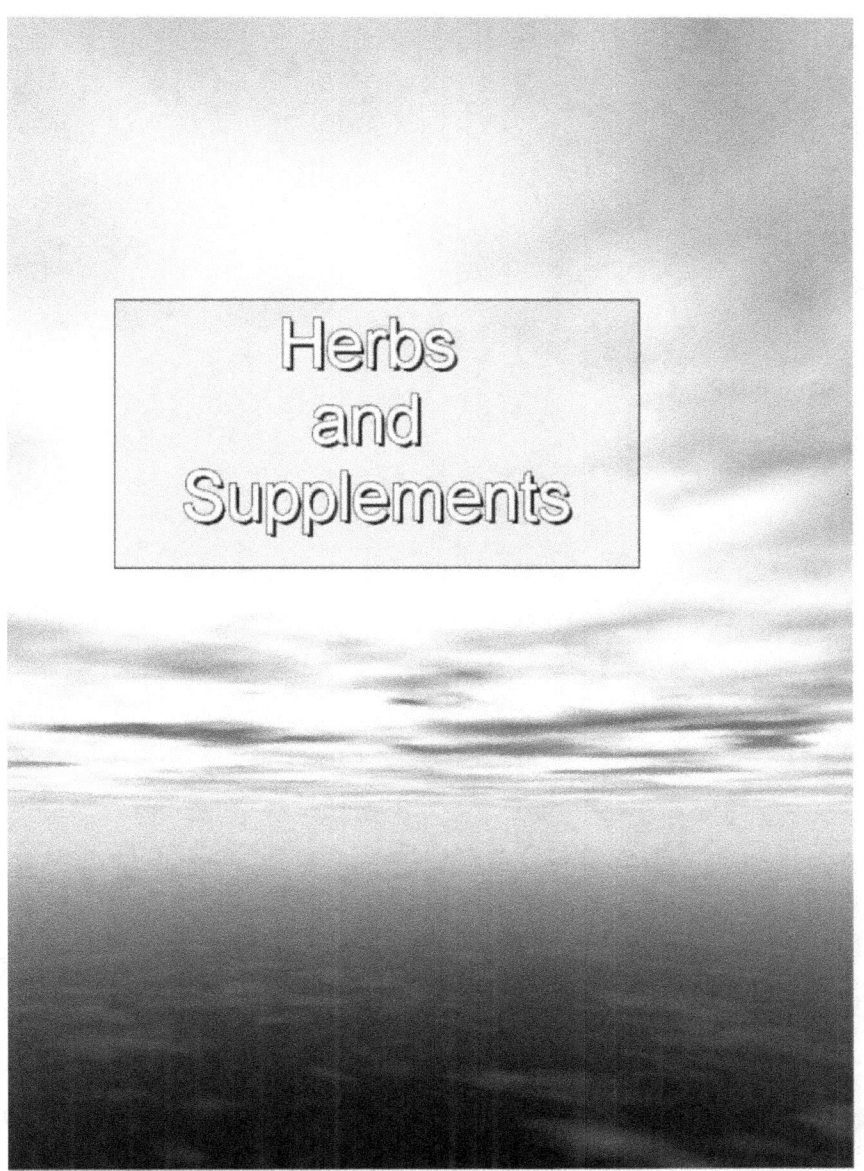

Herbs
and
Supplements

Herbs and Supplements to Support Stress and Brain Health

Herbs, plants, and supplements can support a wide range of all health and health related issues. In this section, we are focusing on three main aspects of herbs and supplements: as the issues that related to Alzheimer's/dementia as we have been discussing. The three areas in major need of addressing are:

- GUT-detox; detoxification
- Stress, anxiety, insomnia
- Clarity-focus/ brain repair

Many of the plants and herbs listed are also known/used as foods, such as garlic. Below is a list of the more common and accessible herbs and supplements. Also listed are some whose benefits make them worth tracking down. Major cautionary aspects are noted, but as always- check any specific conditions against contra-indications, or work with a holistic practitioner or nutritionist.

Also, it is important to note that when you are selecting herbs, and especially spices for health benefits.. avoid the commercial processed brands. Ideally, it is important that the plant has been organically raised, to assure that you aren't consuming toxins, and to assure you aren't missing out on the most potent health-supporting benefits.

These plants-herbs and supplements (two sections) are

not listed in any order of benefit or hierarchy. Nor are they the totality of the possible options. It is enough to get you started, and to get you thinking about alternatives. Tracking down a good herbal reference guide can be a life-changing experience. A few I like and respect, and find very user-friendly are Penelope Ody, and Louise Tenney. You can find their books on Amazon- and used copies are generally very reasonable.

Aloe Vera is fairly common and can be found in many stores and plant shops. If you're lucky, you can find someone and get a clipping, to start your own plant. If not, aloe vera juice/gel is available in health food stores, and in many larger commercial food chains. Or online.

The gel is used as a moisturiser and to soothe the skin. It is also a common holistic treatment for ulcers and digestion. It speeds cell regeneration, and so is a good remedy for burns and dermatitis.

GARLIC garlic is common pretty much all over the world in some form or another. Its properties and benefits are phenomenal. Fresh garlic is one of the most potent and effective natural antibiotic remedies around. Garlic's healing properties come from two separate compounds, which are stored separately in the garlic. When it is crushed or cut... those two chemicals combine. And while the smell of fresh crushed garlic is very pungent-- THAT is when it is most "medicinal." It supports the development of healthy normal GUT bacteria – so is great in trying to rebuild the GUT and digestion.

USES: garlic helps to purify the blood, reduce blood pressure and cholesterol. It possesses antibiotic properties, particularly against candida, and staph infection. It also has anti fungal action. It helps clear phlegm and mucus- so supports treatment of colds, coughs and bronchitis.

It is beneficial as a detoxifying agent, and it can also help to increase appetite.

Marshmallow (the real plant, not the puffy sugar treats:). Mallow is one of several plants that are soothing and demulcent. Because of these properties it is beneficial in helping to treat and heal ulcers and the digestive tract. It is also soothing to the lungs, for coughs. It can also help with insomnia.

Chamomile is a medicinal herb that often grows wild and in abundance. It can act as a digestive aid, and is a very mild and soothing sedative tea, which can help with insomnia.

Tarragon a common herb in many kitchens can be used to help stimulate appetite, and aid in digestion.

Fennel seeds can aid with indigestion, and can help repair the liver following alcohol damage

Licorice has expectorant actions, while also being demulcent and soothing. So it is helpful for treating coughs and colds, as well as support in treatment of healing the GUT and ulcers. It also helps the liver to detoxify drugs and is used for helping treat liver disease. It also supports the adrenal glands, which are important for helping the body cope with stress.

(caution for use with high blood pressure)

Lemon balm the tea has a reputation for supporting longevity. But its immediate use supports relaxation and calm. It soothes indigestion and headaches as well as nausea.

Mints there are many different types of mint, spearmint, peppermint being the two most common. Peppermint is one of the best supports for anything related to digestion, nausea, gas, bloating etc. it soothes the digestive system and helps to break up gas. It can also help by stimulating the liver and the flow of bile. The volatile oil in peppermint is a very specific action for treating ulcers, and therefore helping to heal and repair a damaged GUT

Dandelion the leaves are rich in minerals and vitamins, so are a nutritious addition to any diet. Medicinally, they are an effective diuretic, but is so rich in its own potassium that it does not deplete the body of potassium as many diuretics can. They are excellent for helping to detoxify the blood. The root of dandelion makes a good tea, and can be used as a 'coffee substitute.' It is an excellent liver stimulant that can help with jaundice and rheumatism. It also stimulates gallbladder kidneys and bladder. It also promotes bile production.

Sage oil- protects neurotransmitters.

Rosemary helps stimulate circulation, and is a blood cleanser. It helps tone and soothe the digestive system, especially if stress and nervous tension are an issue. It is also helpful for the liver and it can help to strengthen capillaries/ function.

Ginger Like peppermint, ginger is another great herb/plant for the stomach and digestion. Used in combination- they are great for upset stomachs and nausea/ gas etc.

Burdock the root is an excellent blood purifier- considered to be effective for pulling out deep toxins from the body. It also is an excellent digestive aid, stimulating digestive juices. Great for blood disorders and supporting liver and kidney function, or toxic conditions which need detox. It is amazing for times when the body accumulates too many toxins (as is often the underlying case with Alzheimer'/dementia). It stimulates all the organs that work to eliminate toxins from the body: liver, gallbladder, spleen, kidneys, bladder and skin.

Flax the seeds contain soothing demulcent properties. As such flax is an excellent remedy to support repair of the GUT and intestinal tract. The fatty acids contained in the seeds help to remove heavy metals from the body.

Slippery Elm is almost a cross between an herb and a food, and traditionally has been used as a food, especially for the sick and feeble. It is both tasty and nutritious. It helps to soothe the digestive tract, with its demulcent healing properties. Beneficial for things like ulceration and colitis. The wonderful thing about this plant/tree/food is that it is so gentle that it is safe for even the most sensitive systems. Great recipe to combine slippery elm with healthy yogurt and raw honey- soothe repair and replenish the GUT!

Turmeric strengthens the gallbladder, stimulates circulation, reduces liver toxins, and helps metabolise fats and improve digestion. It possesses non-steroidal anti-inflammatory actions. It also supports healthy joints/function. It also promotes healthy liver function and blood.

One of the compounds in turmeric, which gives it that rich yellow colour, is curcumin. Turmeric can assist your cells by neutralising substances that cause harm, maintaining the cells' integrity when threatened by "stressors," and by providing anti-oxidants to support and protect against free radicals and oxidation.

Turmeric is also recognized as an adaptogen -- helping to support your body against stress and providing immune system support.

Bacopa, or brahmi, is another herb native to India

and has been used for centuries to treat conditions such as anxiety, heart problems, asthma and bronchitis, as well as digestive disorders. It is beneficial for the Alzheimer's patient because it helps both the brain and the GUT. Cognitive specific information in "cognitive support," but noting here that tests have demonstrated significant improvement on retention of new information, and decreases the rate of forgetting the newly learned information.

As such it can support memory and learning. It also promotes calm clear state of mind. And provides the brain with important anti-oxidants and protects the brain.

Aside from its brain related properties, it helps remove toxins from the blood and increases circulation. It reduces inflammation and helps to relieve asthma due to its broncho-dilating properties. It can also support thyroid function and health.

Given its association with improved mental functioning capacity, Brahmi is best taken in the morning.

Gotu Kola a commonly used herb in Indian herbal and holistic medicine. It is a nervine (supports and strengthens the nerves and nervous system). As such it is a good supporting herb for nervous disorders such as epilepsy and senility. Aside from its brain and cognitive benefits (discussed in depth under cognitive support), it helps to strengthen the adrenal glands- which are the organ that help the body process and cope with stress.

Because of these functions, it helps to combat stress and depression, and improves reflexes. It has been used traditionally, to treat a wide range of issues from varicose veins, hepatitis as well as high blood pressure, and more restful sleep. It energizes the central nervous system and rebuilds energy reserves.

It also has beneficial effect on the circulatory system-improving blood flow and strengthening veins and capillaries. .

It also has properties that may make it a potentially useful for treating ulcers. It also has anti-bacterial, anti-viral and anti-parasitic properties. .

- good for fatigue, anxiety, depression

- wound healing, trauma, circulation

- stomach pain, indigestion, ulcers

- anemia, diabetes, asthma

According to pharmacological studies, one outcome of gotu kola's complex actions is a balanced effect on cells and tissues participating in the process of healing, particularly connective tissues.

Ashwaghanda

The name ashwaghanda comes from two words in

sanskrit- which basically translates as" ashva, for horse, and gandha, to smell.. from the horse-like smell of the roots. But it is commonly known as "Indian ginseng."

It is used as an "**adaptogen**" to help the body cope with daily stress. As well as it's support for the brain and cognitive function (see cognitive support chapter), it is also good for decreasing pain and reducing inflammation. It can also help prevent the effects of aging.

Ashwagandha contains many useful medicinal chemicals, alkaloids, choline, fatty acids, amino acids, and a variety of sugars.

Research (over 200 studies on its "healing benefits") demonstrate properties that support:

- immune system protection

- combats stress, helping to balance cortisol (stress

hormone)

- improves learning, memory, and reaction time

- reduces anxiety and depression without drowsiness

- helps stabilizes blood sugar

- helps lower cholesterol

- reduces brain-cell degeneration

- offers anti-inflammatory benefits

In Japan, the Institute of Natural Medicine (Toyama Medical and Pharmaceutical University), has been conducting research into the benefits of Ashwaghanda. They are looking at ways to encourage the regeneration of nerve cells: axons and dendrites in the human brain. This work may prove beneficial both for those who have undergone traumatic brain injury, as well as issues such as Alzheimer's and Dementia, where there is cognitive decline due to the damage to the nerve networks in the brain.

Researchers are noting that ashwaghanda supports significant regeneration of the axons and dendrites of the brains nerve cells. It is also supporting the repair of synapses (the junction or intersection where nerve cells communicate with other nerve cells). The research concluded that Ashwaghanda helps to repair the networks of the nervous system. Other research demonstrated that it supported the growth of new nerve cell dendrites- the portion of the cell that allows nerve cells to receive information from other cells. Finally, a third published study, showed that Ashwaghanda supported BOTH the repair of damaged cells AND promoted new growth as well.

Cinnamon is effective in improving blood glucose control in patients with type 2 diabetes. When taken whole, or in tincture form, it is an effective remedy for yeast infections- particularly those that are resistant to treatment. It is also a good remedy for the stomach and digestion. It can help prevent bloating and gas, as well as nausea.

Additionally, it has been found to help regulate blood sugar levels, and helps to have stable energy and moods. It also has several anti-infectious activities. It can also help relieve pain associated with arthritis.

But cinnamon holds particular interest for neurodegenerative diseases, such as Alzheimer's, MS, and brain tumours. Research shows that it helps to reduce the chronic inflammation associated with these neurological diseases.

Wood Bettony is an excellent remedy for stress and insomnia. It is an effective sedative for children and adults. It is good for helping to treat headaches as well as facial pain. It helps clear toxins and from the blood and opens up congestion in liver and spleen. It is useful for helping to treat liver problems, fevers, jaundice, nervousness, kidneys, neuralgia, pain, lung congestion and insanity. As it is regarded as safe for small children, it is always a good herbal support to have on hand and start with.

Rooibos pronounced roy-boss.. also known as redbush (for those, including myself, that trip over the correct pronunciation:)... is a "tea" from a small specific area in South Africa-- exclusively. Attempts to cultivate it, even in similar conditions, have failed. It beats all other teas for its health and anti-oxidant properties.

Helpful for treating hyperactivity, so can be beneficial for easing the pent-up fidgety energy that often accompanies Alzheimer's/dementia.

One of its best features, is the abundance of the anti-oxidant quercetin- that protects the heart, lowers risk of cancer, helps fight viruses. And it reduces inflammation- the hallmark of almost every chronic degenerative disease.

Two other important compounds in rooibos are aspalathin and nothofagin. Aspalathin helps to balance the hormones and specifically reduces the amount of adrenal hormones. In this way, it helps reduce stress, and it also helps regulate blood sugar levels. Nothofagin has anti-inflammatory activities and along with aspalathin, may help reduce risks of Alzheimer's. Both are neuro-protective.

A high intake of rooibos tea resulted in significant reductions in lipid peroxidation, LDL cholesterol, triglycerides, and an increase in HDL cholesterol levels compared with the control group.

MISCELLANEOUS

Chaga is a hard woody mushroom (sort of)... It has many and wide ranging medicinal properties. Chaga is predominantly known and used as a cancer treatment. It is a potent anti-oxidant, perhaps the most powerful one available, with an ORAC count of 36,000 units, blueberries, in contrast rate approximately 1,500-3,000 units per serving (cup). Chaga detoxes the body, detoxes and helps repair/ restore the liver. Chaga also possesses anti-inflammatory components as well. It is a potent adaptogen, and works to bolster the metabolism to create better energy. It contains hypoglycemic properties as well.

- Chaga is immuno-modulating: it both tones and strengthens the immune system. For auto-immune conditions, it helps to soothe and ease the over-activity of the immune system. But it also has properties that will call an under-active immune system into action.

- Chaga is being used for many cancers, LYME disease, HIV, hepatitis, liver conditions, as well as supporting diabetes, detoxing the body (blood, intestines, and liver). Chaga is being incorporated by highly respected cancer facilities, such as Sloane Kettering, and Cancer Institutes of America! I have known cancer patients who have used it in their treatments and as support for traditional protocols- and it kept the body from "crashing" during treatment.

- It is a surprisingly tasty beverage, usually consumed as a TEA. It is mild enough to be tolerated, even by young children. It is also "neutral" enough in its flavour to combine well with a wide range of other herbs or "flavourings." It combines well with cinnamon, cloves, vanilla, rooibos, orange, cocoa. it can be combined into coffee cocoa or other beverages.

- Chaga also bolsters the metabolism and has many other health properties, helping the body to create its own energy and adaptogenic, coping with stress.

- Chaga has tremendous benefits as liver-supporting, detoxing and repair of damaged liver. It is also a good blood detoxifier.

Blue-green algae: is considered a superfood. It has amazing nutritional value as well as health-enhancing properties. So it is both a "food," and a supplement. It contains plenty of the amino acids such as isoleucine, luesine, lysine, methionine, tyrophine and... tryptophan (the feel-good turkey chemical:). Thus providing important proteins/ building blocks for healthy bones tissues and organs, as well as neurotransmitters.

It also contains choline, Bcomplex, magnesium and a whole host of other healthy nutrients.

It can help strengthen the immune system, in part by helping the body create interferon (a component of the immune system).

It increases oxygen in the body.

Apple cider vinegar ask anyone in holistic circles for a remedy- and chances are that Apple cider vinegar is high up on that list-- no matter what the issue. It seems to be something of a cure-all. Especially a good "raw" unfiltered brand. It is especially rich in potassium, and all the minerals that were in the apple. It is great for cleansing impurities out of the blood, and for reducing calcification in joints and just improving overall health.

One of the effects: of vinegar on blood sugar levels is perhaps the best researched and the most promising of apple cider vinegar's possible health benefits. It is also rich in malic acid which gives ACV its anti-viral, anti-bacterial and anti-fungal properties

Honey

Honey is one of the better sugars for the body. Ideally sugar for Alzheimer/dementia patients should be minimised. But a little honey can be very beneficial, and can help with some things like sleep.

Honey also possesses antiseptic and antibacterial properties. In modern science we have managed to find useful applications of honey in chronic wound management. It can also help boost the immune system and can minimise seasonal allergies. It is also one of the best remedies for soothing coughs.

Raw, organic honey is loaded with vitamins, minerals, and enzymes which protect the body from bacteria and boost the immune system. Cold and flu symptoms, such as coughs, sore throats, and congestion are also kept at bay when treated with honey.

Honey also possesses antiseptic and antibacterial properties. It can also help with indigestion, as the antiseptic properties of honey relieve acidity in the stomach. It also neutralizes gas. This is probably why honey and ginger work so well together;) Another potential benefit of honey, is for the liver. Optimal fueling of the liver is central to optimal glucose metabolism during sleep and exercise. Honey is the ideal liver fuel because it contains a nearly 1:1 ratio of fructose to glucose.

Probiotics: We talked about probiotics under foods, in yogurts, and kefirs etc. But probiotics can also be taken as a supplement (capsule form). They can help to reestablish the healthy bacteria in the GUT. The GUT possesses healthy bacteria, which are essential to maintaining good digestion and health. The GUT also has small amounts of "bad bacteria," that we acquire through various ways, and poor diet. The healthy bacteria are essential to keep the bad bacteria from overpopulating the GUT. They can be especially helpful in times of stress, or when we have been given a course of antibiotics (which kill ALL bacteria, even the helpful GUT ones). But stress can damage the healthy bacteria, and so can poor diet, as well as mental and physical factors.

Enzymes protein-like substances that are formed naturally in plants and animals. They act as catalyst (speed up) the digestive process in the body. They occur in raw foods. When foods are cooked, the natural enzymes are destroyed. This is why it is essential to include lots of fresh raw foods in the diet. There are 4 main types of enzymes, each of which specifically targets types of foods we eat. Lipase- breaks down fats. Protease- breaks down proteins, Cellulase- breaks down cellulose and amylase- which breaks down starch.

Enzymes also help with detoxing the body, by helping to release and remove toxins through the colon, kidneys; skin and lungs.

SUPPLEMENTS

ALA: alpha Lipoic Acid ALA helps metabolize sugar in the body, especially in muscles, where it supports energy metabolism. It also supports nervous system health. It is considered a valuable "universal antioxidant" because it is effective in water-based substances such as blood, while its reduced metabolite, dihydrolipoic acid (DHLA), is effective in fatty tissues and membranes.

Recent research indicates that it can restore T cell function. (a type of white blood cells, a key part of the immune system). They are essential part of adaptive immunity. ALA is also a powerful chelator for heavy metals- meaning it removes them from the body.

ALC acetyl-L-carnitine- is an amino acid derivative, meaning it is made from l-carnatine (One of many amino acids in the human body/diet- amino acids are the building blocks of proteins). Human clinical studies of this compound are currently underway, and the early evidence from animal trials is encouraging. Many people take ALC as a cognitive enhancer.

It can help increase energy production in the mitochondria (the energy-power of all cells), helping to boost both physical and mental energy. As a supplement, it is often used to help improve memory, it also may slow age-related mental decline that is not associated with Alzheimer's. It may also help to protect the nervous system.

Taurine Calming Neurotransmitter. It is a crystalline, free-form amino acid. It is a soothing,
inhibitory neurotransmitter and plays a major role in stabilizing the heartbeat and electrical activity of the nerves. Taurine is often called the most important amino acid you've

never heard of. This is because it was once thought to be a non-essential amino acid, meaning that the body could produce it. But this is not the case. It can be created in the body from methionine, or from cysteine in the liver, but vitamin B6 is needed in order to do this. And children cannot make taurine at all.

Taurine is found in the heart, skeletal muscles, white blood cells and in the nervous system. When the body is under stress, or exertion, it does not produce the needed amounts of taurine. Another reason why it is so important to reduce stress-- the body doesn't function property under stress.

Taurine also helps to remove toxins from the body. It helps to protect the liver cells from oxidation, ensuring that the liver can remove toxins from the body safely.
It can help improve nervous energy, such as anxiety and ADHD. It also supports optimal brain function.

Taurine helps to control the flow of calcium into and out of the hearing cells in the ear. These properties may help to prevent progressive hearing loss and may also be invaluable in the control of tinnitus.

It can also support the body during exercise, to have better stamina and work harder. It also helps to remove lactic acid from muscles, which allows them to work longer.

GABA

Promotes Relaxation & Mental Focus Clinical studies have shown GABA helps increase the production of alpha brain waves to create a profound sense of physical relaxation while maintaining mental focus. GABA is synthesized directly from glutamic acid. It has an inhibitory effect on the firing of neurons and supports a calm mood

GABA is an amino acid known for its importance in nervous

system functioning. It is an inhibitory neurotransmitter, naturally produced in the brain, which counters excess brain stimulation. This formulation provides Free Form GABA to promote optimal absorption and assimilation. It promotes relaxation and supports the nervous system.

Nattokinase

Is a traditional remedy for diseases of the heart, and circulatory system (cardiovascular disease) for hundreds of years. Nattokinase has the distinct ability to break down the adhesive substance that makes arterial plaque very sticky. In this way, it supports a preventative and reversing effect on blood clotting and plaque build up in the arteries. It also has blood-thinning properties so should be used with caution by anyone on blood-thinners.

Nattokinase can also break down unwanted toxins, cleanse

and detox the blood, and clear away undigested proteins in the gut, and helps stabilise a healthy GUT. It has the distinct ability to breakdown peptide bonds and liberate amino acids. It is being studied for its possible role in treating cancer.

It may help to stabilise blood pressure, and it aids in preventing blood clotting, and it helps dissolve existing blood clots. It dissolves fibrin and helps the body to keep blood vessels clean and healthy. It may also help prevent heart attacks and strokes. *It is also distinctly noted for its ability to cleave the amyloid plaques in the Alzheimer's brain, and help to remove them.*

N-acetylglucosamine (NAG). This naturally occurring enzyme helps repair the mucosal lining in both the stomach and the intestines by aiding in the synthesis of the viscous top layer of the gut mucus.

Lglutamine- another amino acid... it's amazing how potent some of the simplest things can be:) one thing it is great for, is curbing sugar cravings. As such, it also helps alcohol cravings as well (alcohol is a sugar:). It also does a lot for healing the stomach and GUT. It helps treat ulcers and "leaky GUT" syndrome (where toxins leech from the GUT back into the body). It also helps the body to repair ligaments, tendons and cartilage. This is the same property that makes it the fuel for the small intestine, and therefore boosting immune function (most of our immune system is in our GUT).

It can also cross the blood-brain barrier, so it is able to provide glutamic acid to the brain, which the brain uses as fuel.

HCL   is hydrochloric acid. It is the digestive juice, or fluid, formed in the stomach to break down food. If you don't have enough stomach acid to break down food, all your careful (and expensive) supplementation and meal preparation will be ineffective. As well as all the other functions of stomach acid, one of the important things it does.. is killing off pathogens (bad bacteria, yeast and microbes) that come into the stomach. Without enough stomach acid- those "bad bacteria" can come in and set up house-keeping in the intestines/GUT.... and that's bad for the good bacteria and healthy immune system and digestion.

Also, stomach acid begins the process of protein digestion. The Pepsin in our stomach begins the process of breaking down protein. It also helps to pull minerals out from our food, so they can be absorbed. Without enough stomach acid, we cannot get the needed minerals from our diets. Also, the stomach acid stimulates the pancreas. The pancreas can then secrete enzymes that help with digestion. If the PH in the stomach is not optimal... then the small intestines can be damaged (leaky gut).

Stomach acid is necessary for absorption of many nutrients and vitamins, such as B12, magnesium, zinc and Vit C, among others.   It is also important in the activation of enzymes, hormones, and neurotransmitters

Huperzine A. Also known as Chinese club moss, this natural medicine works in a similar way as Alzheimer's drugs.   But more evidence is needed to confirm its safety and effectiveness. Traditionally, it has been used to treat bruises, muscle strains, swelling, rheumatism, and colds; to relax muscles and tendons; and to improve blood circulation.

It has been found to cause increase in levels of acetylcholine, one of the chemicals that nerves use to communicate in the brain and elsewhere in the body.

Choline Neuroscientists have been studying the potential of choline to prevent cognitive decline and the onset of Alzheimer's and dementia. It is also being looked at for its potential to regrow brain cells as we age. In studies, phosphatidylcholine was found to stimulate the growth of new brain cells and neural connections ie, neurogenesis. It plays a role as a key building block of cell membranes, which means it protects the cells that line the digestive tract AND the liver, as well as brain and nerve cells. Phosphatidylcholine can lower cholesterol, protect the liver from disease, including hepatitis, and appears to help alcoholics stave off cirrhosis.

Similar to this is

PhosphatidylSERINE (PS), which is being used for treating Alzheimer's. It helps protect against age-related decline of mental functions. It also improves thinking skills in children and is used for treating ADHD. It can also help treat depression and cognitive ability. . Early studies, though promising, were based on cow-derived supplements. It's not known if plant-based phosphatidylserine supplements offer any benefits.

PS, is part of the cell structure and maintains cell function, especially in the brain. It is a naturally occurring lipid (lipid=fat) that is makes up cell membranes. It is a brain nutrient. It may improve cognitive function in healthy brains and help reverse cognitive decline.

Phosphatidyl Serine and Taurine: These natural anxiolytics work to increase dopamine, relaxing the central nervous system.

Theanine can be found naturally in green and black tea. Theanine helps to relax the mind, soothing or diminishing the desire to have an adult temper tantrum. Theanine is a non-essential amino acid that can be absorbed across your brain. It is also a natural phytochemical found in Japanese green tea. As a supplement, it supports the mood centers in the brain, and a calm, relaxed mood. It increases the brain's alpha-wave activity (alpha associated with relaxation). Higher alpha waves are also associated with greater mental sharpness. In other research, it increased feelings of relaxation by 40 percent among people with serious behavioral disorders. Bonus: doesn't cause drowsiness.

SAM-e All living things contain SAM-e. The body makes SAM-e from mathionine (an amino acid). However, levels of SAM-e can vary, and they can decline, due to age or other factors. It helps with over 35 biochemical reactions that involve enzymatic transmethylation.

Methylation process is the mechanism by which the body rids itself of potentially damaging compounds, synthesizes neurotransmitters, makes components of cartilage, regulates enzyme activity within the cell and maintains the flexibility of cell membranes. It can help promote healthy joint function, and also supports mood and emotional well-being.

5-HTP is a precursor to serotonin, a neurotransmitter involved in sending messages through the nervous system. It helps support a healthy nervous system. Clinical trials demonstrated its effectiveness in the treatment of depression.

It is a natural appetite suppressant. And some evidence indicates its ability to help treat headaches, and fibromyalgia. Also, 5HTP can cross the blood-brain barrier, where other chemicals, like serotonin do not cross as readily.

Be sure to buy high grade good quality 5 HTP..and equally true for all vitamins and supplements. Food based vitamins are best-- but shop around for a good quality source. There are some wonderful places online where you can get reasonably priced, good-grade supplements. **Vitacost**.com is a great resource--- but there are plenty of others, as well.

Herbs and Supplements Guide and Worksheet

On a Scale of 1-10 I would rate my comfort and experience of herbs and holistic approaches as _____

Were you surprised to find many familiar foods, spices and herbs listed, that are also highly medicinal and helpful? _____

The nearest health food store or co-op is _____ (look it up:)...

Which local supermarkets have the foods I might like to try?

Does my market carry any organic brands?

Two herbs I might try for healing the GUT are:

1._____

2._____

Two herbs that I might try, for detoxing the blood:

1._____

2._____

Two herbs I might try, for detoxing the liver:

1._____

2._____

Two herbs I might try for stress:

1._____

2._____

Two herbs I might try, for mental clarity and focus:

1._____

2._____

I was most surprised to learn:
_____
_____
_____

Two supplements I think might be most helpful (to start with).. are:

1._____

2._____

I can try to find these at: my local health food store or co-op____? My holistic practitioner____?
Online at Amazon or a vitamin site____?

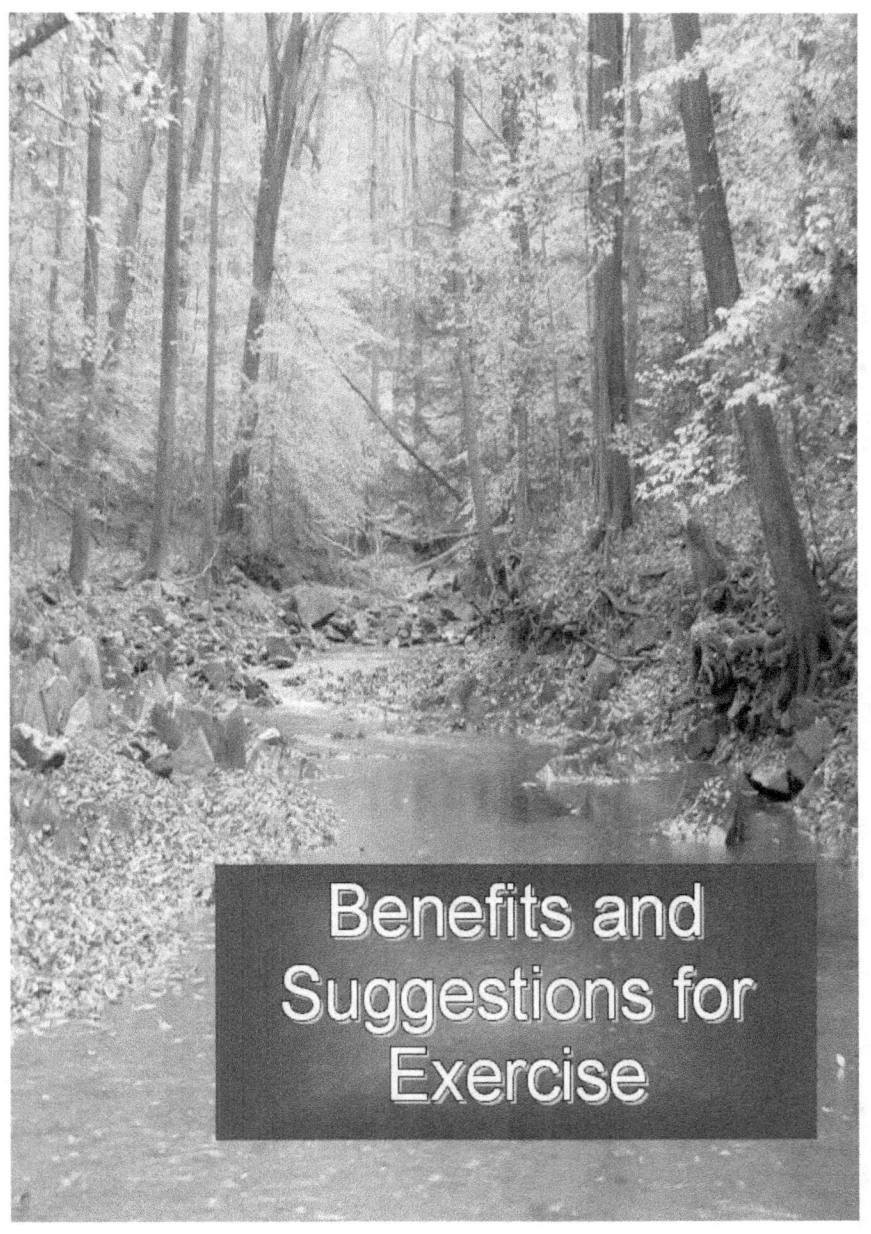

Benefits and
Suggestions for
Exercise

Benefits and Suggestions for Exercise

We all know that exercise is good for you. And we know exercise is important in order to remain healthy. It keeps our bodies functioning optimally. Getting the blood and fluids in the body circulating, helps it do its various jobs. Our muscles and joints get better nutrients, which helps them remove toxins and maintain suppleness and strength. When our blood circulates, all the organs, including the brain, receive nutrients and oxygen. Also, the other half of exercise's benefits: that good circulation is good house-cleaning, finding and removing toxins and waste. Exercise is for the body, what housekeeping is in the outside world. It makes sure everything is where it belongs for optimal functioning, and removes the dust, dirt and debris.

As we age, especially if we are not already in optimal health, we tend to slow down. With Alzheimer and dementia patients, this is often even more true. As the brain struggles against the challenges of memory and cognition- more and more things get left by the side of the road. Just as though you/ they were hiking, carrying a heavy pack. They hike for a while, and as the hiker tires, they may decide to drop the least necessary items. This makes the struggle of hiking against fatigue... a little easier, and allows the hiker to proceed toward their destination. The same is true for Alzheimer, dementia and cognitively challenged patients. As their condition progresses, the brain is more challenged, it "tires" more easily- literally and metaphorically. So it puts down the less essential items: non-essentials.

These non-essentials include information and memories, but also- any activity or task that is not performed regularly, or hasn't been performed in a while. Although, ironically, often with the aging brain, the oldest memories are deeper and stronger. It becomes "harder" to learn new things.

But this doesn't have to be the downward spiral of continuing decline and loss that it often becomes. Just like any person who is out of shape... a fitness program - both literal and metaphorical- can begin to turn things around, especially when it is combined with good nutrition. Alzheimer and dementia patients are no different. Granted, there are different challenges that accompany working with this population. But for them, exercise and activity are MORE important, not less.

Exercise increases circulation, especially to the brain. Activities can stimulate the brain into processing-- and any/all processing is a bonus for the challenged brain... new connections can be made, new pathways built.

The trick when working with the Alzheimer or dementia patient is twofold.

First, it is important to accommodate emotional and cognitive limits and stress-levels. Start slow, keep it short, and pay attention to the "limit," or saturation. Know when they are "done," and either create break-time, or leave it until the next day/ time.

Secondly, is making sure the brain is as prepared and ready for learning as possible. This entails making sure that the brain is getting as much of the vital nutrients, vitamins etc that it needs-- just like a child we send to school. We want to make sure they are fully nourished, so that they can get the most out of their learning.

Secondly, and this is more specific to the Alzheimer and dementia patient or client: and that is removing the toxins, and providing as much supplemental support as possible. In this way, the support is giving the brain as much chance as possible, for rebuilding neural connections and creating new pathways.

Eliminating as many toxins from the brain and body as possible is crucial. Just like giving a car a complete tune-up and oil change... so that everything runs as smoothly as possible. With the Alzheimer/ dementia patient... foods, vitamins and supplements can support focus, and combat the "stress" they may feel when exposed to and experiencing "new" things. Diet and Nutrition, combined with exercise will minimise the brain-stress of processing. It can also help the brain to be ABLE to make neural connections (removing plaques), and repair axons, dendrites etc (see previous chapter on detoxing the body).

Anyway- with all of these things taken into consideration (and even without), even the moderate to severe Alzheimer/dementia patient can become accustomed to exercise and activity: looking forward to it, enjoying it and reaping the benefits.

WALKING

One of the easiest activities is walking.   Ideally walking unassisted is the goal- as this supports an optimal upright posture (CRUCIAL for balance and safety)... Ideal posture for walking, or standing: the shoulders should be lined up so that they are over the hips-- look at the person sideways. Often, in older people- you can clearly SEE this forward tilt.

They are hunched and learning forward. This will accentuate more and more, over time. It is BEGGING for accidents and falls. As it progresses and the balance decreases, they begin to reach out to hold onto almost anything. This is the first step of a downward spiral and an accident/fall waiting to happen.

When assisting an elderly person to walk... it is beneficial to NOT HOLD THE HANDS, and guide them forward!!!! Even though in the MOMENT, it might be the most expedient and "comforting," over time it is creating a catastrophe in waiting. As they become acclimated to the comfort of "holding onto" something... they become more and more insecure without it... and begin reaching for things to "hold them up."

Ideally, when helping them to walk....walk BESIDE them, with a hand or an arm, under the UPPER arm, just beneath the armpit. You can use this to maintain and support an UPRIGHT position and posture. You can also FEEL and sense their balance, and gently guide them in one direction of another.

If it is necessary to hold or support the lower arm, hold UNDER the forearm, above the wrist. If a patient is used to hand-holding, it may take a little while for them to become used to a change. BUT, it is important to break the dependence on the hand-holding. They quickly grow accustomed, and dependent, on holding onto SOMETHING... and they will begin to look for things to hold them up, that may not be stable and suitable. Plus, they will stretch and reach for something to HOLD, often bringing themselves OFF balance in the process. This combination of unsteadiness and poor balance can contribute to falls and poor movement. If they don't feel SAFE and emotionally comfortable walking or moving-- they are going to become more and more stationary and sedentary.

I have found that Alzheimer patients crave and cling to familiarity and routine. This can be a challenge when first starting something new. Using walking as an example, they may become uncomfortable, begin making excuses I need to cook dinner, or other diversionary statements)... use diversion and distraction and a small goal. Let's walk up to that flower (something that might catch or hold their interest). Or perhaps walking up to a familiar destination. 'Let's walk up to the store on the corner." Or your grand daughters house, etc... Try using distracting conversation.

The second day, repeat the same route/routine. You should find each day is a little less resistance, as they, and their brain, knows what to expect. Once a walking route is established, try to lengthen it. Initially there may be a resistance as the usual "turnaround" spot is passed, and it may be necessary to employ the same diversionary tactics as with the initial process. But once the activity is "established," lengthening the distance or duration is easier. The pathway is there... so it is just a matter of minor modifications and "strengthening."

When I am walking a patient/client. I generally like to see them begin to BREATHE. They will pause, as though to "catch their breath." And if watching, you may/should notice visible breathing. Not that you want them panting and out of breath... but this increased breathing supports the oxygenation of the brain.

Often, I discourage the use of a walker for short distances or around the house, when there is supervision. ALWAYS stay on the side of safety and if no one is around, make sure they have a walker or cane, if they need that support.   When walking as an exercise, even with someone to watch and help them, the walker can be a good support mechanism. They can then use their own sense of exertion, and have a ready support when they need to pause for rest.

In the good weather, it is ideal to find an outdoor location to walk.   Fresh air and sunshine are vital to health and well-being. If that is not an option, mall-walking is a good second choice, especially in rainy or cold weather.

In some instances, treadmills may be an option.   But they won't give the added benefit of new visual sensory experience to engage the brain in the activity. And they won't offer the fresh air, and scents and stimulation of being outdoors, or even in a mall.

Water walking "swimming" aquasize

In early to moderate stages- it would be great for the normally healthy-fit person to try water based exercise. Being in the water is soothing, on body-joints and mind. There are more and more pools, often local state colleges, which have community-based programs. Voc-rehab centers probably know of places and programs. Most of these pools are what is referred to as arthritis-rated- so the water temperatures are considerably warmer than the typical public swimming pool. These temperatures are geared toward seniors and rehab therapy.

For the more advanced cases or for people who are not in good share, or 'brave." There are water-walking options that offer a lot of benefits as well. Walking in the water is the equivalent of three times the walking-time on land. Plus, it doesn't stress joints- as the water is buoyant, taking weight off the body.   So, walking for 20 minutes in the water, is the equivalent of walking for an hour, on dry land.   For patients who are less stable, they can walk along the shallow end of the pool, holding onto the rim/edge.   Having someone walking next to them, offers support and reassurance.

For a patient who is less sure and stable: again, think long term.   Don't push for instant success.   If they are wary, judge their levels.   Maybe just visiting on day one.   Or sitting on the edge with their feet in the water.   Most pools, especially those that have programs, have good steps with railings, or ramps or supports to help get in or out of the water. And remember, they often take their lead from their caregiver-mentor.   So remember to be calm, relaxed and soothing.   Soft encouragement and increments can create tremendous long term results.

Exercise classes, yoga

I have been working closely with one moderate-advanced Alzheimer/dementia client (not entirely sure which her diagnosis is:)... for about a year. One of the things I started her doing/ doing with her... is a class that is very common in Vermont, called "bone builders." I am not sure if this is available nationally/internationally. I highly recommend this for anyone who is interested in staying healthy, but doesn't necessarily want the higher impact exercise programs. It IS, or can be, a workout, although low-impact, and each member decides what level they want to work at. The programs are all volunteer run, and free to participants. There are no membership fees or obligations to go non-stop.

For most of the class members, it is a led series of exercises and they follow the exercises and participate to varying levels. With the Alzheimer patient, I act as something like a physical therapist or occupational therapist-- not in terms of a profession... but in that, I mentally modify whatever exercise the group may be working on. And I guide her, physically through the motion. If it is raising the arms above the head. I stand behind, gently holding the forearms, by the elbows. This way, she can see and watch the rest of the class performing this action.

I gently lift her arms up, sensing limits of her range and ability. Each time, I can see the range and suppleness increases. Additionally, once she has an "idea" a repetition-imprint, she, or her body... participate more and more. She will randomly comment, and often it is incoherent "babble" talk, or just inconsequential. The group is very supportive and embracing of who she is. This in itself, is very comforting for the patient.

The first few times attending, her attention and stress kept the class time short. But each time she was more comfortable, and made less and less "time to go" inferences. Within 2-3 weeks

(2x/week), she sat through the entire hour, participated to various levels in ALL of the routines, and was very happy and "engaged." The entire class often offers feedback, and all of them noticed the changes in her mental and emotional states in just a few weeks. She was markedly "better," on all levels, including cognitive and communication.

Yoga is another low impact class. And there are classes in chair yoga. I have had several discussions with yoga instructors about working with this population. Absolutely in the early stages, it has decided benefits for calm, clarity and overall "happiness" factor. I have not seen or done this, as I do not have access to the environment/ setting, but I believe a similar mentor-support could be done with yoga or chair-yoga. For a yoga class though, I think it would need to be a specially designated class. In the exercise class, and bone-builders, outbursts and chatter are not a distraction in most instances. In a yoga class though, the other members are there for that peaceful ambiance, and might find ongoing distractions annoying.

But there are many other organised low-impact exercise programs and many of them can likely "accommodate" around the unique needs of the Alzheimer/dementia populations. I highly encourage caregivers and family members to investigate this possibility. Especially if there is a full-time paid caregiver- work that into their responsibilities. And, as the patient is in better spirits- it is a tremendous relief and ease for the caregiver. Remember, what benefits the patient/ client, also benefits the caregivers.

Activities

Research is coming in that **SINGING** has tremendous benefits for Alzheimer/dementia patients. It seems to help cognitive function, health (breathing) and happiness-well being. Singing groups, which perform songs from the well-known musicals and other easy to follow/remember songs. Many groups incorporate hand and arm movements to encourage the physiological/physical element. And like exercises, each week, songs will be reinforced. Singing uses a different area of the brain, which is also good. The more areas that engage... the more the stressed areas get to "rest," and... the chance to create new neural connections and wiring. And again, there is the social aspect.

We are social creatures. We LIKE (most of us), to participate in groups and group activities. This can be especially true for our seniors, who feel more and more marginalised. A volunteer singing group could be formed through a local community center, senior center, or even a church group. All it needs is CD's a CD player, and a volunteer to lead the group. Again, remember, especially for the more moderate to advanced stages, it may have to start in small increments and build up:)

For those who still have a stronger cognitive function, engaging them in as many activities as possible is ideal. Reading, or reading to them (this is even good for advanced patients. A reading group is another possibility.)...knitting, quilting, especially if these are skills they have had life-long.

Playing cards, checkers, and bingo. Anything that is done socially, is within their range of abilities, and uses cognitive function. This falls more under cognitive support, than exercise-- BUT, it rightly belongs in both categories.

For men, maybe putting a golf ball into a cup, if they used to be golf players. Horseshoes, beanbag toss... there are so many possibilities to keep them engaged and active. It just requires the modification of awareness re mental, emotional and cognitive state of mind. Over time, ability and participation can and will improve.

Exercise and Activities Guide and Worksheet

Are there any activities you/ your patient participate in regularly?

1._____

2._____

These activities help to support what aspect of an Alzheimer support program?
Social _____Cognitive____ Physical health/fitness_____ Stress relief _____

It would be good to add activities that will support the different aspects of a support program:

Which areas are not as fully addressed:

Social_____ Cognitive _____ Physical health/fitness ___ Stress Relief ____

some activities or exercise programs I/we/they might add into this program might be:

1._____

2._____

3._____

4._____

What are some activities you/your patient has done during their life? Long term, or short term?

1._____

2._____

3._____

4._____

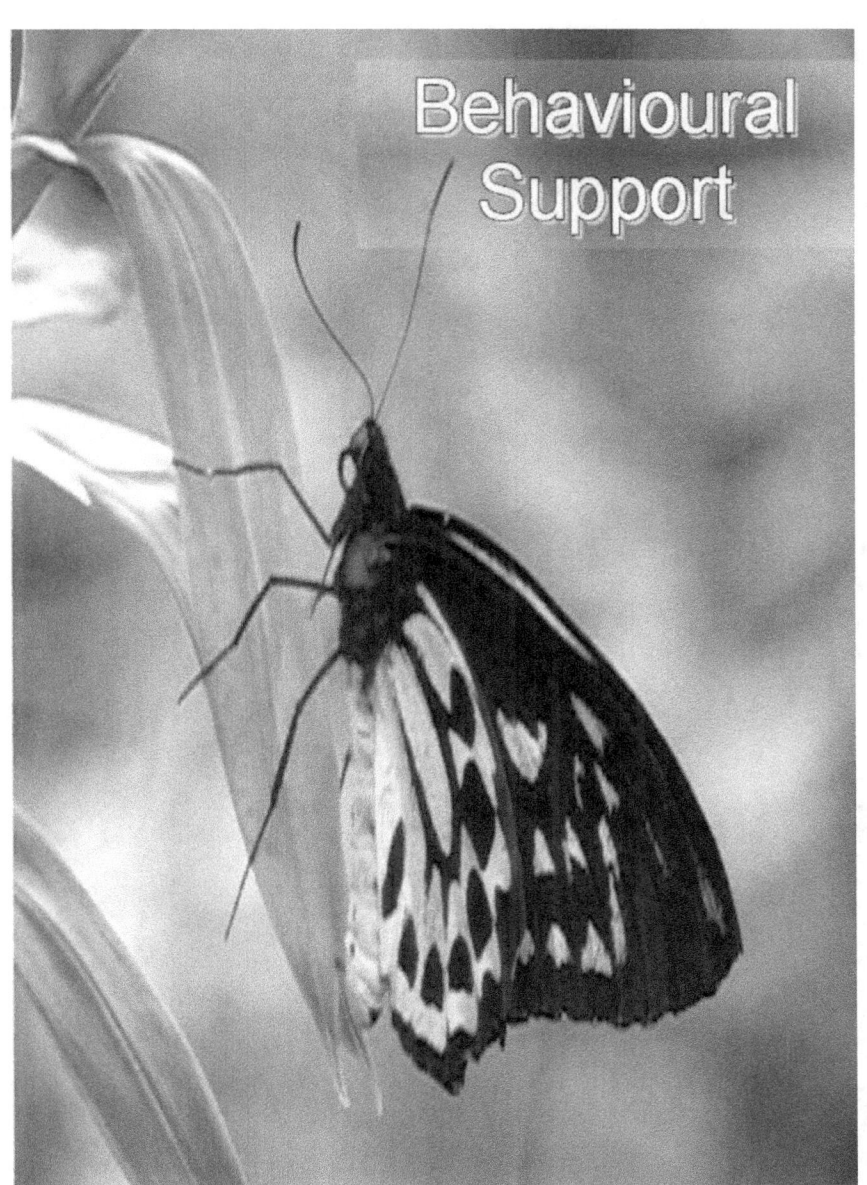

Behavioural
Support

Behavioural Support

Often it seems like the Alzheimer-dementia patient is unstuck in time... this is especially true the further they advance in the progression of the disease. Their conversation or chatter, will wander over vast spans of time. Often culminating in a burst of sadness, tears, or "regret."... It is difficult to know if the sad emotions stem from the associated memories, or from some sense of detachment they "realise" at some intrinsic level.

Often, even the more severe patients... **know...** something isn't right... they will say... I can't get the words out, or ... something to the effect that parallel to the entire jumble of thoughts, memories experiences and emotions.... is a part or layer... of awareness. This has to be the hardest part of any degenerative disease or condition- especially that affects the brain or mind.

Watching the decline of Alzheimer's patients/ clients often reminds me of the book/movie Charlie/ Flowers for Algernon. In this story a severely mentally retarded man is a prime candidate for an experimental procedure. This surgery results in tremendous brain growth, and he becomes one of the most brilliant scientists in a relatively short period of time. Tragically, it turns out that the changes do not hold, and the second half of the story is watching him, as he watches himself decline. He is completely aware of what it taking place, and utterly helpless to stop the digression, and fighting against his cognitive decline. Ultimately, he is left where he started in the beginning of the story.

While the early stages of Alzheimer-dementia are often unrecognised... there must be a stage where a person knows... that they are forgetting more things, losing more things or becoming confused. Far more than is "normal," even for the aging process. And of all the things we could lose, the loss of our memories, our autonomy and more crucially, our "self" must be the most terrifying journey anyone could have to take. And this is not a journey of choice. That must make it all the harder... it is an enforced journey without a happy ending.

I often see deterioration of mood, when a patient is tired, brain-stressed, or hungry. This is why it is so crucial that any program address all aspects and components of health. Exercise, diet-nutrition, and cognitive support.

Honour and Respect their desire to be Present

I will often see a patient trying to communicate, or participate and become angry because they cannot contribute. Often, two or more people may be talking, and the Alzheimer patient will become angry and frustrated: they have been "Jabbering" but the other people continue talking over and around the person. They become angry, because to their mind... they have something to say, combined with the all too human drive and need to participate and be included. They are, essentially, being ignored. And they know it.

If any "normal" person was being edged out of a conversation, they would also, rightfully, become annoyed.   I have often found, that just taking a moment to acknowledge and respond to the Alzheimer patient, soothes them and strokes them. It is comforting and calming for them to know they are there.   They are fighting the biggest battle around "being present." How must it feel then, when all too often, they are treated as though they are decidedly not-present?

So it is a good rule and practice, in regards to moderate to advanced patients/clients... to acknowledge and respond. Just like small children, who will often want your attention at inopportune moments... so to with the elder or Alzheimer-dementia patient.   Just because their speech doesn't make sense, or is "chatter," doesn't diminish their genuine desire to make connection, communicate, or be acknowledged. Sometimes it is worse-harder, since they expect to be given respect and attention, and they are losing that vital component in their life.

In terms of the chatter-talk... often I will find in their desire to communicate, or connect verbally in some way... that they will come out with odd or random statements. Often a non-committal or reassuring response is all they need. The point is to determine if there is something important they "need" to communicate and can't, like- the need to go to the bathroom, for example. In other instances though, it is the desire to communicate, or have reassurance. Often responses like. Really? Maybe later, etc-- while they feel a little "cheap," in the moment... serve a greater good than trying to decipher what may not make any sense to begin with. It may be emotional-based/driven communication, rather than physical-present based communication. They want-need to be acknowledged or reassured, so finding the appropriate response serves that purpose.

Also, as their condition deteriorates, and their world, literally, grows smaller... their script... becomes more limited. Meaning... chances are they have a number of routine-related questions, comments and thoughts. Just the way they may have emotional-memory of people they know... they may not have distinct names for each person that they know.

One patient generally uses her daughter's name when asking for something, calling for 'someone" or in distress. She does know her caregivers... but generally not by name. When one of her caregivers is on duty, the woman will call her daughter's name when she wants or needs something. She is not distressed when not-daughter appears, and is generally reassured/comforted when told her daughter is at work.

Soothing a conversation with a Response - Closure, rather than an answer

One of the things I have found, again, in regards to the more advanced patients and clients. Often they will ask a question, or engage in conversation that doesn't seem to have a goal.

I have found that rather than going to great lengths to determine if there is a genuine need or question: sometimes it is far easier to have a few rote responses that can give closure to their potential distress. Asking them questions to try to figure it out.. can sometimes make them more frustrated. "It's all good." with a reassuring tone can often be a far more successful engagement, and cause a lot less stress and frustration, all around. In this sense, they have a closure to the "conversation," that may not have had any necessity, and it soothes their need to feel that they are safe and okay.

Sometimes, regardless of the best of intentions, there are outbursts and spikes of emotion. I sometimes find this, for example, when trying to get a patient to do something like helping into the bathroom. Or into and out of the car. In other words, doing something that is difficult for them on SOME level- either physically, neurologically, or emotionally.

And sometimes it is just a "rant" that self-escalates. Remember, in many ways, they are living in their own little worlds. What they experience mentally and emotionally may have absolutely nothing to do with what is going on in the present. Patience and soothing are the best tools.

Sometimes, I will do nothing, and let them have their moment. Like a small child, they may be tired or frustrated and allowing them to work through it and not interfere is the "path of least resistance," as well as honouring where they are at. If a mood or behaviour becomes excessive, it can help to have a way to get their attention. Often when I see the fist-shaking, I will hold the wrists and call the person by name, sharply-clearly; as a means to get their attention. Not as a punishment, but more as a way to bring them "back" to the present, here and now... which does not hold any antagonistic input... and reassure them, it's okay. It's good. If I think they have the capacity, I will also ask... what do you need? Thus giving them the option to communicate and respect their needs and wishes.

Ground Rules

There are a few of what I call ground rules. "No biting." is a clear and understood rule. I convey this with one particular patient/client.. not as a punishment, or a confrontation, but more as a reminder.. much the way you might remind a spouse or partner to put the dishes in the sink/ dishwasher.... as they are about to walk away from the table--- without them:)... in that instance, you might clearly call out "dishes," as a reminder to the departing spouse/partner.

This kind of neutral reminder tone can be very effective when dealing with an escalating emotional state. I have one patient, who will raise her hand toward her mouth as her frustration grows.

Now, she tends to pause and stop... KNOWING I am about to give a sharp-clear reminder of NO BITING." I have found that I can extend this rule to the silverware. Often as she decides she doesn't like something or is just being difficult, she will open her mouth, annoyance clear... and then bite the spoon in a sort of petty/ childish anger.

This "rule" has also been beneficial one time when she was angry about something (getting frustrated trying to get out of the car, and hitting a neural logjam).. and she opened her mouth as though to bite me. I know that this is not uncommon in patients, especially as they are in the more advanced stages.

Breaking a rant by changing the tone- sometimes when a patient gets snippish or mean or sad or angry etc... I will respond as though they had just said something very happy or pleasing.   REALLY???? expressing-conveying pleasure or pleasant surprise. I have been amazed, at how often this will shift them out of their previous state. They will answer me with a "why yes, of course" kind of tone and response-- immediately shifting tone and mood. Remember, there isn't a strong short term memory function. USE this!

A few things that tend to benefit better behaviour and minimise the outbursts

It is important to remember, outbursts are often a neural

response as often as emotional ones. This is why it can be helpful just to "sharply" call their name-- just to shift the brain away from whatever it was jammed and stuck behind. Either neural or emotional, shifting the brain-attention away from whatever had them "jammed up," can be an expedient and kind approach. When possible, I also try to make eye contact, and get them to focus on what I am saying... Again, this is something that can become "easier" with time and repetition: as they and the brain learn.... when they see/hear/experience **A**... then B follows....

Routines are very helpful and beneficial. When someone is in a routine, the brain doesn't need to figure out what is going to happen next, or what is expected of it, or what it needs to do. This is why we form habits, so that we can do things by rote. If we had to learn something again, new, every time we did it-- we would quickly be exhausted and frustrated.

Also, sometimes, like with meals, it can be beneficial to consider outcomes over expectations. With one patient, the family is concerned with her weight. She can sit at the table for a certain amount of time, after which she will just get up. If pressed, she will try to insist there is something that needs to be done. In other words, her brain-attention has reached its saturation point. If pushed, she will become more resistant, and nasty. Getting her to eat when she is in this frame of mind is unsuccessful.

Instead, especially when she is not having a "good day," I will often cut up her food into finger-sized manageable chunks, and leave it in her "path." Often when she is in a restless mood, she has specific behaviour patterns. One of them is fussing by the sink, and repeatedly peeking out the window (she may have been somewhat of a busybody in her earlier years;)... SO, rather than trying to get her to come to the table, or relax and settle down, I will leave the plate on the counter, near where she is fussing.

Sometimes I can get her to take a bite, if I come up and say... "hey, try this," as though it is something newly cooked and it is a "treat." Occasionally, once she begins to eat, she will be more ready and willing to cooperate. Other times, it is important to just know... it isn't going to happen: and pushing the issue will only cause an escalation. Again, leaving a meal where it is accessible, can serve the same purpose.

Often, with this more advanced patient, she will begin to eat with her fingers, making quite the mess of it all. But, she is eating. Some of her caregivers have an issue with this... but it seems that the woman prefers to feed herself, no matter the associated mess. She generally will eat more successfully this way. And often, she will reach for spoon or fork as she becomes more clear and focused on the task.

And as with other things, when sitting down to a meal, on a

daily basis, she becomes more accustomed to the "idea" and "habit" as an expectation and known practice.

Diet and Nutrition can play an important role in mood and behaviour, as was discussed in the chapters on nutrition. So, often when I see escalated and frustrated behaviour, my first questions are: what has she been eating, how did she sleep? And following that, I ask how much exercise and activity she/he has had.

Again, the reminder, that if the frustration levels are high-- crank up the turkey, sweet potatoes, and lentils... or any of the other "happy foods" from the list.

Problem Solving

Also, it can be helpful to figure out if there is something "legitimate" that they are focused on or agitated over.

I had one client who repeatedly was trying to go outside. This was a little unusual, and it was consistent and persistent. I finally figured out there was a piece of paper outside... that I had put aside as unimportant... and they were very adamant that they wanted this piece of paper. Once the paper was in hand... the escalation and frustration subsided, and no further attempts to "escape."

So, sometimes they legitimately want or need something that they either can't convey or can't convey successfully. It can be a little like charades, or trying to communicate with someone from a foreign country... a bit of guessing and intuition play a big part.

Exercise

Exercise can be another great asset in behavioural support. It helps the body feel more physically comfortable as it gets to move around and gets blood circulating. That blood flow will also help clarity and cognition. The brain needs fresh oxygen and nutrients... Exercise and blood flow help get those to the brain. Also, think for a moment how you might feel when you have been cooped up or sitting idle for too long. The human body really wasn't designed to be sedentary-- certainly not to the degree that we live, in modern society. We sit for hours and hours, at desks, at tables, at the computer and at the television. Getting out for fresh air, a walk or other exercise... is soothing to body and brain. It removes that nervous energy-- because we USE IT UP.

I have a client that I take out for exercise and errands. When I come to pick her up she is fidgety and antsy. Up and down, here and there, fussing with things-- sometimes imaginary. When she comes home, she is able to sit, relaxed and comfortable, watching television for the rest of the day or evening. I have found that her caregivers will come in and ask who has had her for the day, or what has been done with her. When they are told that I have had her or taken her for the day, they are like "YES!" because they know she will be calm, she will eat better, and ultimately, she will sleep soundly through the night.

Another important aspect of behavioural support for the Alzheimer-dementia patient is the **vitamins and supplements**. Relieving stress, and supporting cognitive function. There is a whole section on that, so I won't go into it again, other than to re-state that it can make a huge difference in increasing their well-being, by lowering their stress-levels, frustrations, and anxiety.

Ultimately, using a range of strategies, including diet-nutrition, and exercise, it is possible to manage daily routines so as to keep a pleasant and happy patient who is engaged, and at a deeper level, even if they can't express it: they have a sense of well-being.   Their life is a little richer, and fuller- which encourages them to WANT to be present, and help "bring them back," much more successfully than if they are left to sit around, and decline into a fog of oblivion. They may not be the whole person they were prior to the onset-- but they can regain a lot of who they were, and discover new things as well. But it is a concerted effort that all involved must be on the same page, and working toward the same goals.

Behavioural Support Guide and Worksheet

I notice that I/ my patient tends to become agitated or angry when:

_____

_____

I have found that this helps to bring them back to a calmer state:

_____

_____

_____

The next time they are upset or angry or sad, I might try

_____

_____

_____

Do you keep any kind of food journal? This is a handy reference to check and watch for corresponding behaviours and moods. Granted, sometimes- because they often live in a world of memories that wander randomly-- their moods just happen, regardless of what we do. But this is why it is so important to keep the brain in optimal health: to support them staying present, grounded on all levels in the NOW.

Managing behaviours strategically: maybe you notice there is a particular time or circumstance that creates difficulty more than others. Maybe it is getting a shower, or feeding/meals. Consider what strategy might work to minimise the agitation. Example- maybe they are calmer after exercise, so timing and scheduling a problematic issue in such a way that they are most likely to be "agreeable."

One of the most troubling behaviours they experience is:

_____

_____

I see this behaviour the most when

_____

_____

One possible strategy for avoiding this problem might be:

_____

_____

A Simple Guide for Tracking Foods, Moods and Behaviours

	Mon.	Tues.	Wed.	Thurs.	Fri.	Sat.	Sun.	Comments
Irritant Foods								
Beneficial Foods								
Exercise and Activities								
Vitamins-supplements								
Sleep Pattern								
Inciting incidents								
Level of clarity and well-being								
Comments								

You can either list items separately, or maybe total them up. At first it might be helpful to list them down. This way you can keep track of which foods are included, and figure out which ones are most helpful

irritant foods

_____

_____

beneficial foods

_____

_____

Exercise

_____

_____

vitamins-supplements

_____

_____

sleep pattern

_____

_____

inciting incidents/experiences

_____

_____

It can be very beneficial to keep a moderate journal or track what is added or taken out of the diet. This way you can begin to determine what things contribute to problematic behaviours, and what changes might be helping them to feel and function better. This is why it can be easier to introduce changes a few at a time.

Otherwise, you can be left guessing which ones worked and which ones might be less helpful.

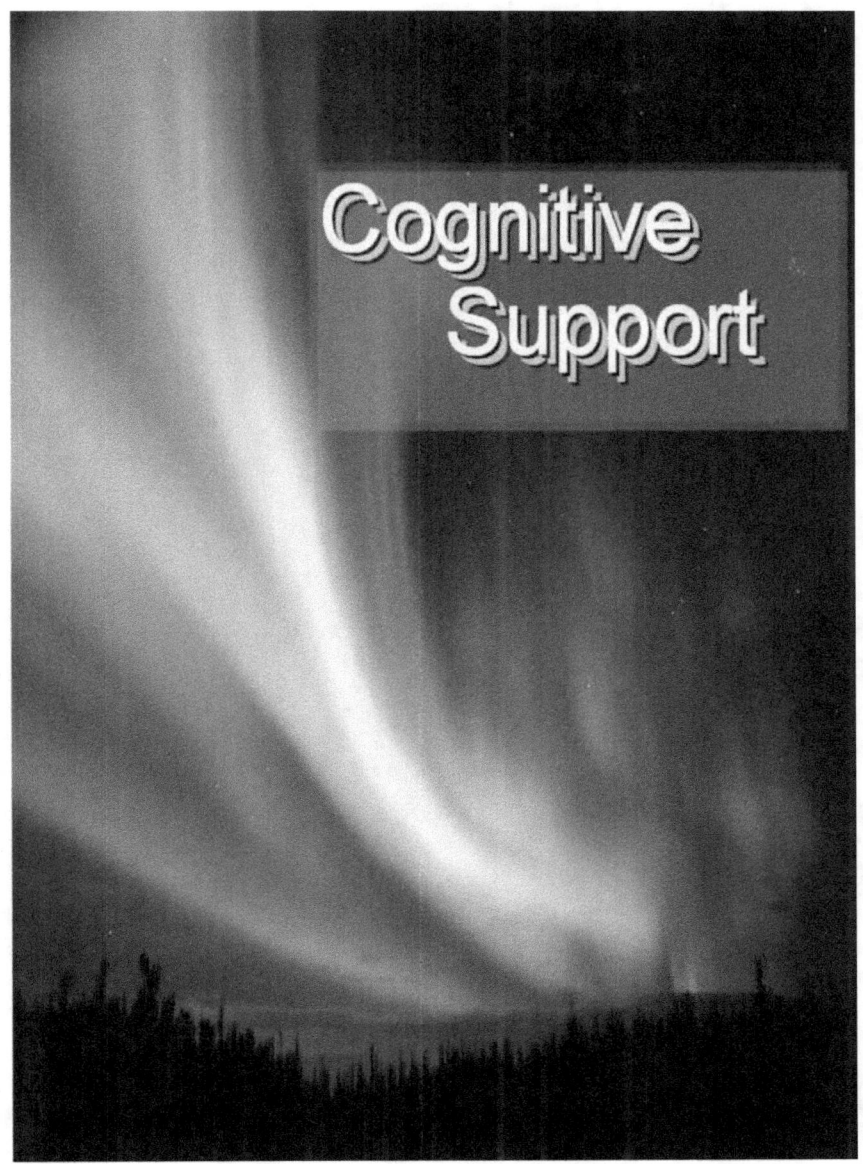

Cognitive Support

Cognitive Support

In creating a program that gives maximum cognitive support for the Alzheimer/dementia patient, two aspects need to be addressed: both **diet-nutrition**, and **external stimulation, activity and exercise**.

It is vital that the brain has all the **maximum nutrients** it needs, and **minimal toxins** to interfere with processing. Additionally, in order to rebuild or sustain a healthy brain- **exercising the brain** with mental challenges and "**data retrieval**," are crucial. The brain, in this regard, is like a muscle, and needs to be kept in shape. To do this it needs exercise. Exercise for the brain, is thinking, experiencing new things. Experimenting. Working things out. And as noted earlier... data retrieval.

Data retrieval even in small increments, builds and strengthens pathways in the brain. Answering simple questions, so long as it requires "thought." can be very beneficial. Questions that can be answered in simple yes-no... feigned agreement... may *not* be as beneficial. If the brain is challenged or can't figure something out, they are unlikely to inform you, they have no idea. Instead, they will often feign agreement or disagreement. Oh yes. Of course. And No. These kinds of answers may not be accurate indicators of information. Are you cold? Asked once, may be of course, yes. Asked 10 seconds later, may get a no.

Granted, some questions, like being hot or cold, may have no alternative frameworks. But many situations CAN be shifted away from yes-no, into something that gives a more accurate insight into need or brain processing. Is this red or blue? Do you want chicken or fish? Who is this in the picture? What are the names of your children/ grandchildren, etc..

Starting with information that they should know/ remember..

develop the pathway and get the brain used to digging around in its memory-files. And.. getting it back out... maybe even asking, point to your son, dog, or whatever, in the picture... if the speech is not there.. at the moment. The information may be.

For the more agile Alzheimer's mind, I will go into more detail on activities and things that can be helpful afterward.   But I did want to preface the importance of making sure the brain gets food, oxygen, and practice...

The brain is a magnificent structure. It only weighs about three pounds. But those three pounds oversee everything that keeps us alive, allows us to function and interact with the world around us.

The cerebral cortex alone- the front part of the brain where we process thought/ ration... contains over 200 BILLION neurons and 125 TRILLION synapses. Neurons are connected by thousands of synapses, to each other, neurons communicate through AXONS... like the pipe cleaners that connect tinker toys. A neuron is like the HUB... the axon is like the long sticks that bind and hold them together.

Information, nerve impulses, flow down the axon, to a neuron-- where they "jump" across to another neuron-- via neuro-transmitters. Neurotransmitters are like chemical carriers... that "ferry" the nerve impulse across the "gap" between neurons... bridging the space inbetween.

The brain uses up to 20 percent of all the energy/ calories used up by the human body. It uses glucose (a simple sugar) as its energy source.

When we consider feeding the brain, note that it is also important that we have, or are, detoxing the body, and supporting healthy digestion and absorption. Otherwise, the nutrients, vitamins and supplements... will have a harder time getting where they are needed- or, might not get there at all. Remember, the brain uses a large percentage of our calories and energy, but it needs the rest of the body to receive, break down, process and transport those nutrients and energy TO the brain. Like a car, the engine might be the most vital part, and the most expensive... but without tires and brakes, steering and oil pump, water pump etc...the engine will just break down... or won't be able to take us anywhere:)

Supplements that support Cognitive Function

There is no particular order to the listed supplements and suggestions. Nor is this a complete and total list. It lists things that appear to be most beneficial, while also posing the least "risk factors." And as always, I recommend doing homework, and ideally- working with a holistic practitioner and/ or nutritionist to construct an ideal regiment that will have optimal impact and outcomes.

Information on these supplements is in relation to brain/ mood and Alzheimer's specifically. This does not list other properties and benefits, as that would make a very lengthy list and wander away from the main goal of supporting cognitive function. Many of these items are covered in vitamins and supplements. The information here is as it specifically relates to the brain and cognitive function.

Taurine: is an amino acid, often referred to as the most important amino acid you've (we) never heard of. Our absorption of this amino acid, like many things, tends to decline as we age, so supplementing with this can be very beneficial. It is a calming neurotransmitter. It is a soothing inhibitory neurotransmitter. It also stabilises heartbeat and electrical activity.

GABA- supports a calm mood. It helps increase alpha (relaxed state) brain waves, supports physical relaxation, and mental focus.

Astaxanthin- is an anti oxidant, and more importantly, it is a lipid (fat) soluble antioxidant. As a free radical scavenger that is 65 times more powerful than Vit C as an antioxidant. It is able to cross the blood-brain barrier and protects the brain from oxidative stress. It is used for treating Alzheimer. It helps support strength, stamina and endurance.

ALA- alpha lipoic acid: can stabilise cognitive function and may slow the progression of Alzheimer.

Chaga (mushroom)- stimulates metabolism in the brain tissue, but calms the nervous system- in other words... it isn't a stimulant in the same way caffeine is. It is more like it promotes optimal function.

Rooibos/ruibos/redbush: aids in lipid peroxidation in the brain. It contains both nothofagin also demonstrates significant anti-inflammatory activity and, along with aspalathin, may help to reduce the risk of Alzheimer's disease. Both appear to protect nerves. "protects the brain & nervous system against a process known as "lipid peroxidation".

This process occurs when damaging free radicals attack nervous tissue and brain cells, resulting in destruction of the protective outer layers of the brain cells, which leads to cell death. Over time, the damage accumulates and can lead to degenerative brain diseases like Alzheimer's.

Bacopa aka brahmi- supports cognitive function, encouraging a calm relaxed state of mind. It contains chemicals that enhance the function of neurotransmitters ability to stimulate dopamine (the happy feel good chemicals).

Gotu kola: is a rejuvenating nervine (tones soothes and helps repair nervous system). By promoting restful sleep it helps the brain and body do their work of detox, clearing and releasing stress. It helps stress and depression. And balances the nervous system. Rats tested with gotu kola had retention rates as high as 60 times higher than untreated rats.

Ashwaghanda: is an adaptogen. It combats stress and improves cognitive function. It improves learning and memory. It reduces brain cell degeneration, supports significant regeneration of axons and dendrites (the mechanisms of "communication" in the brain). Reconstruction of synapses. It boosts healing of damaged nerve cells as well as new cell growth. In studies done in dementia induced rats, treated with ashwaghanda, within 21 days the rats were observed to be in "learning mode." when the brains were studied, new axon and dendrite growth was observed.

Cinnamon: possesses two compounds that appear to inhibit "tau" proteins that accumulate and create the nuerufibriliary tangles, inside the neuron cells.

Coconut oil: Studies indicate that Alzheimer patients have a hard time using (utilising?) glucose in the brain. The disease is sometimes referred to as diabetes of/ in the brain. The ketones in coconut oil can serve as an alternative source of fuel. Coconut oil does possess less ketones than other sources, but it lasts for up to eight hours. Studies indicate it seems to help about half of Alzheimer patients. Note, there was no data to indicate the stage of progression, or if any of the other holistic or nutritional supports were in place.

The brain doesn't get enough glucose-- but the monolauric acid from coconut oil... is a good substitute. The essential fatty acids and the fact that the fat in coconut oil converts into lauric acid- which feeds the brain and nerves. Studies have shown cognitive improvement over time, taking approximately 3T serving/daily. Some studies are indicating cognitive improvement immediately after eating coconut oil.

Omega oils, in particular the omega 3's-- which we do not receive in adequate supply. Reduces inflammation and is a "brain food." The omega oils are commonly found in the form of fish oils.

Krill oil is a particularly good source for the omegas. Krill is a crustacean (like shrimp), and as such is a much more sustainable source for the oils. It can be cultivated with greater ease. Also, krill contains other beneficial properties as well. It is more readily absorbed and utilised by the body than the fish oils. It is high in vitamins A and E. It is a powerful antioxidant.

The astaxanthan that is unique to krill oil, may be able to handle multiple free radicals at the same time. (caution advised if allergic to shellfish). There is some belief of a connection between low level of omega 3's and cognitive decline, loss or memory and thinking skills. Researchers have been testing if krill oil supplements can improve brain function. Researches in Norway found rats performed better on skill tests. They also found it produced similar affects to anti-depressants.

Nattokinase: nattokinase is a supplement derived from Natto, a process of fermenting soybeans (remember, fermented foods very beneficial). It is mentioned here because it does cleave the amyloid plaques that accumulate in the brain and interfere with neurons....plaque which inhibits learning and memory. And because it can also improve energy.

It contains a proteolytic enzyme that has fibrinolytic health benefits. It helps to rejuvenate healthy fibrin metabolism and reduce blood clotting --also break down unwanted wastes such as toxins, cellular debris in the blood, and undigested proteins in the gut. With the distinct ability to breakdown peptide bonds and liberate amino acids, (read supplemental cautions, re coumadin, vitamin K, clotting etc if you have any blood-thinning issues.)

Niaciniamide: Researchers gave mice the equivalent of a human dose of 2000 to 3000 milligrams of niacinamide, and the results were shocking. "Cognitively, they were cured," the head of the study claimed "The vitamin completely prevented cognitive decline associated with the disease, bringing them back to the level they'd be at if they didn't have the pathology." Niacinamide also improved memory in mice without Alzheimer's.

Cannabis oil: more and more research is being done around medical marijuana, and the powerful healing properties of cannabis oil. Research indicates that it may trigger anti-oxidant cleanse, removing damaged cells and improving the efficiency of the mitochondria (energy source that powers the cells) Studies link cannabis to neurotropic factor, which protects brain cells and promotes new growth.

Activities

As mentioned earlier- good food and supplements are a vital component of keeping a healthy brain, and of rebuilding brain health. The other element of this is Exercise. Mental exercise. Get the brain working. Dust off the cobwebs, open the windows and get fresh air and sunshine in. literally and metaphorically.

There are many exercises and activities available, at all ranges of skill and ability. The goal is to incorporate them into a regular routine. Try to re-establish any old activities or hobbies, as well as introducing new ones. New experiences are great for the brain. Plus, you never know what your patient might find as a new interest or skill.

Bingo has long been a hobby of the elderly. However- it actually is a wonderful cognitive exercise. Bingo entails hearing and visual crossover. A player hears a number, needs to visualise it, look on their card for a match- based on auditory information, and engage in the action of marking the correct spots. It is fun, social and helps keep the mind sharp.

Playing cards, also engages the brain. And depending on the game being played, it can also challenge the memory- remembering what cards have already been used, or if someone else might have certain cards. And card games can range from the very simple, to the very complex and many inbetween.

Board games, for the social stimulation, plus varying degrees of mental exercise based on the game. It might just be moving pieces around the board, like in Parcheesi, or solving a mystery such as in the game Clue, or a crime-solving game. In today's market, also-- with the advent of computerised games... it is probable that many games could be played without other human players.

Crossword puzzles, word searches and jumbles. Simple to complex... keeps the brain nimble and thinking.

Knitting, Quilting. Crocheting:

Many activities like knitting, actually involve a high degree of brain function. In fact, in some progressive educational programs, they teach the children at a young age, how to knit and crochet. They do this because it develops the brains math-centers. Knitting is all about pattern and repetition... but it is essentially a kind of "numbers." It also keeps dexterity sharp, as the hands have to perform the intricate motion.

Hobby kit: from bird houses to picture frames that need painting. Senior years can be a journey into new activities. Remember Grandma Moses? Get a painting kit (paint by numbers)... or clay, an airplane kit... there are so many things that can be done, and are packaged in a way to make the process easy to follow and accomplish.

A drawing/painting Art class. It doesn't have to be good. it just has to be fun/ enjoyable. . Creative activities might not engage the cognitive functions as much a other things.. but it does engage the brain, especially the creative side-- which may be less taxed as it is not as involved in most of the challenged cognitive functions.

Little chores around the house: maybe folding laundry, or if you are folding laundry, give the patient the hand towels to fold... or sort socks... (all depending on their stage of decline)... also, if it is a task they are used to performing, determines if it might be in their deep memory. Sweeping the floor or wiping off counters. Generally, the more advanced patients have a shorter attention and focus... and do not stay "on task" for too long... but all of it helps. And over time, it will build on itself and there should be improved outcomes.

Stimulation, new experiences: research shows that whenever we have a new experience, our brain engages... processing new input. Without over-stimulating, or stressing.. it can be good to take Alzheimer patients/ clients/ family members to new places. Maybe a walk in a different mall or park. Or a different restaurant for lunch.

Cognitive Support Guide and Worksheet

What percentage of our daily calories does the brain use?

_____

What is the brains primary fuel source?

_____

What is a secondary/alternative source of fuel that the brain can utilise? _____

List two herbs or supplements that promote calm and relaxation:

1._____

2._____

and note where you might be able to locate them to add to your protocol

List two herbs or supplements you might try that will help improve cognitive function:

1._____

2._____

An activity that might be good to try, or bring back into practice

Do I know someone who already does this or can give me additional information? If not, where-how can I find out more about where this activity might take place, times and schedules?

_____

Activities that can be incorporated in the home might be:

1._____

2._____

3._____

Caregiver Support

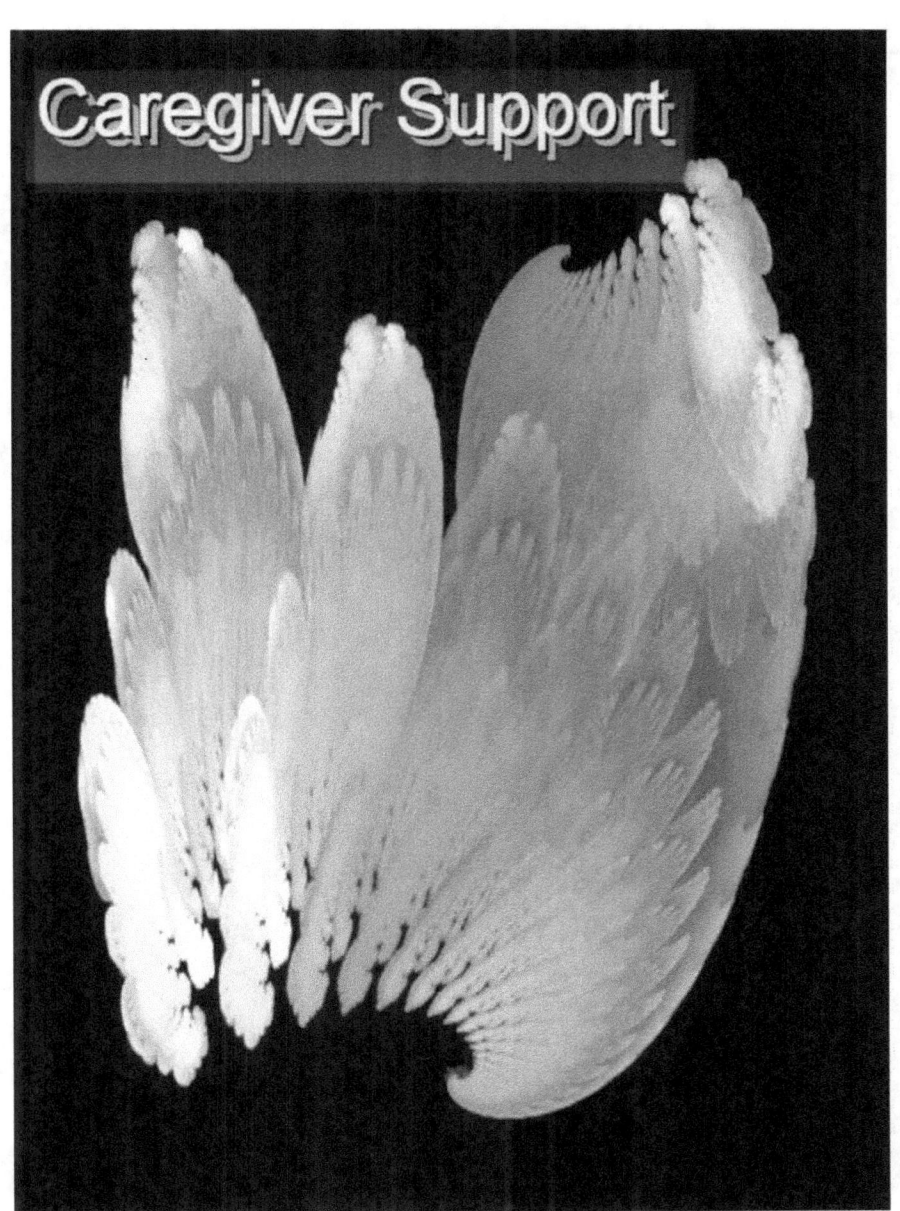

Caregiver Support

We know the health statistics of caregivers. The drain and depletion of caregivers own personal and health resources is excessive. More than sixty percent of Alzheimer/dementia caregivers rate their stress as high, or very high.

Caregiver Statistics:

- Thirty percent report symptoms of depression.

- Caregivers have an additional 9.1 BILLION dollars in health care costs, over non-caregivers.

- The stress and drain of care-giving is NOT IMAGINATION!

Generally, caregivers will experience/have:

- poor eating habits
- sleep deprivation
- don't exercise
- don't stay in bed when ill
- postpone of or fail to make medical appointments for themselves

- increased risk of depression

- increased risk of alcohol, tobacco or drug use

- increased likelihood of chronic illness
- more likely to be overweight, high blood pressure and/or cholesterol

The daily routine for the caregiver is exhausting. A massive amount of mental and physical energy is spent anticipating needs, addressing every moment, overseeing non-stop, and running interference between the world and the patient.. diverting outbreaks, cleaning up messes, soothing upsets and emotions that do not eve have a clear causative agent.

In many ways, it is more exhausting than child-raising.. as children are learning how to communicate, and their cognitive function, while still developing.. is healthy. I know that when I am working with a patient/ client... I am at optimal for 5-6 hours, depending on the client, state of mind, and the amount of "drain."

But there is a limit to how long I can decode, decipher and

engage on the other side of babble-conversation before my brain and energy starts to feel depleted. After that, I know I am not at my best, and have to be more conscious and conscientious about patience, tolerance, and taking a breath. I need to watch myself to make sure I am engaging from a good, relaxed and calm frame of mind. The longer the duration, or if it is several days in sequence, the more taxing it becomes.

So for the primary caregiver, this stress and drain is monumental. Especially given the general nature and temperament of the typical caregiver. It can be even harder, when the caregiver is a family member. There are long-standing behaviour patterns, ingrained- both good and bad. Also, the struggle of watching a parent in decline adds a tremendous amount of added emotions.

Often the personality of the caregiver is such that they suppress or neglect their own needs and health...perpetually giving their energy, time, resources and emotions into their care-giving/ patient. This is one aspect of my own training that I really appreciate.

In the Andean spiritual teachings I was taught a very powerful distinction between western cosmology and "religious paradigm," and the Andean indigenous perspective. In western mythology- the collective underlying belief is that we are all fallen from Grace. As such, the western-modern psyche is perpetually on a quest for redemption, forgiveness and absolution. We must have forgiveness BEFORE redemption. Confession comes before communion.

Alternately, the Andean teachings, while Christian in their daily beliefs, still carry the older teachings which keep them closer to the Earth, and how to maintain physical, emotional and spiritual balance. In their original cosmology- they have no "Fall from Grace." They were never kicked out of the garden. As such, they still have an intimate connection to their natural environment, in a way that western modern life has lost.

But the part of their teachings I found the most interesting are based on that subtle distinction. Since they were not born into "original sin," they are not born in need of redemption. As such, in their practices, while they truly and deeply live and practice, balance and reciprocity-- they believe that they should always fill and replenish themselves first, before giving. In this way, they give from a place of fullness, which does not deplete the self. And as such... they are able to give more fully, deeply and completely.

Much of this book and training, focuses on the Alzheimer patient/ client/ family member. The reason for this is because the focus IS on the patient. As it should and needs to be. The caregiver needs support. The patient needs healing, treatment and physical care.

But also, it is essential to help the Alzheimer/dementia patient.. by doing everything and anything to make their life easier, to help them be more functional, improve their cognitive functions and minimise the stressful behaviours. And by doing this, by helping the patient/ family member to be as healthy and functional as possible...this supports the caregiver as well. If you don't improve their function, you can't improve the caregiver's role and plight. In this regard, what serves and benefits the one, benefits them both.

Since so much of the information in this book addresses stress, this information is equally beneficial for both patient and caregiver. Foods that relieve stress for the patient are good because they relieve stress. And Stress is stress is stress. So those same modifications will benefit the caregiver as much as the patient.

Emotional-personal balance:

Journal- put your thoughts and emotions down on paper. For really high stress days... try this. Write the Bitch-session.. all the horrid nasty terrible selfish things you want to say, or are feeling. No holds barred. Whatever comes up, write it down.

You may note that you feel better just for owning and venting the thoughts, and giving a voice to unvoiced, un-acknowledged emotions. NOW, take the bitch-session, and let it go. Burn it. Tear it into tiny pieces, and burn it, or flush it....take the symbolic act of releasing the negative emotions. Honour, them, but ultimately, they are harmful to you. So don't hold them. Sometimes, my teachers would then suggest writing a thank you, gracious letter, as a follow-up. On the same person/topic/emotion/situation. This can help shift that negative destructive energy into something wiser, smoother, more peaceful.

Keeping a journal, can also be a way of monitoring your own levels though, over time. You can learn to see your trigger points, and see and learn to prevent the cliffs, and crashes of your own. Maybe you will learn to notice that several nights of poor-sleep are a precursor to losing patience with your Alzheimer's patient. It is a good way to be able to step back and monitor patterns, so that we can gain insights into our own processes, and maintain ourselves optimally.

Have a confidante, bitch-buddy... This can serve the same purpose. Just a place to vent, without judgment or recriminations. Maybe someone who can offer insights or input. Maybe have a confidante that can be relied on like a AA sponsor... giving the hugs and support and replenishment, when you are depleted.

Grounding and relaxation techniques, prayer, meditation etc... Going out for a walk, especially away from the noise and bustle can be very soothing. Go sit against a tree. It sounds crunchy, but it works. Just sit back and try to feel the slow patient compassion of the tree, which has stood in one spot for years, watching it all go by.

Breathing- huge benefit. When we are stressed or concentrating, we forget to breathe, or to breathe well. Take a few slow deep breaths into your belly. Close your eyes. Ten breaths. You can even do the breathing when you are driving (but not the closed-eyes part;).

There are many guided relaxation tapes, dvds etc. They work for a lot of people. And again, can be used when driving, or with earphones when shopping... when falling asleep at night.

Physical balance:

Exercise: alternative to smoothing out the wrinkles of stress...

is the approach that says burn it off. Go out and do something that requires exertion. Not necessarily excessive- but enough to get body working, a light sweat maybe, but definitely to raise the heart-rate. Shoot baskets, run a few laps or blocks, try the climbing gym. Recruit a friend to try something totally new. Maybe a dance class, or a sport/ activity.

Diet-nutrition

It is just as important for you, as it is for your patient or client. Remember this. If you aren't at your best, on all levels, you aren't able to give your best, do your best work etc. YOUR body also needs support and maintenance. Many of the supplements and suggestions are for stress. Make a list of a few that you can try yourself. It can also give you valuable direct-experience of their use and benefits, which will further help the well-being of your patient or client.

Good Sleep

If all the other components are in place, then you should be getting restful and replenishing sleep. It is as vital for you, as for your patient. There are supplements that can help support good sleep. But ultimately, each person needs to find out their own best routine. Some experts will advise to turn off all distractions and learn how to quiet down and "train" yourself for bedtime. This may work for some.

I personally find that listening to a story on tape, is like getting a bed-time story, to which I fall asleep more readily, and without chasing the days thoughts around and around in circles. A few minutes of stretching, or yoga, breath-work or a meditation-exercise can help shift the body down into "quiet mode" or "night-time" mode... But do try to find a way so that you don't fall asleep with the caregiver wheels and worry wheels spinning round and round. Because very often, you will find you wake up, right where you left off.

Mental balance:

Find you-time. Write, read, draw, colour. Anything that is recreational, has no parameters, doesn't tax the brain, and you can immerse yourself in rewarding-escapism:)

Have a social outlet: an online support group, join a new activity, take up a hobby.

Take breaks. Planned time off daily-- even if it is 15-30 minutes while a patient is napping or eating. Spend that time stretching, yoga, exercise, or creatively... In other words... devote the majority of mental and physical attention to yourself (within safety parameters)... and worry less, for a few minutes, about the moment to moment needs of your patient/ family member.

Support groups, live or online.

Search out caregiver support services. You might find local or church volunteer groups that can offer respite to a full-time family member caregiver. Insurance may cover respite care to give a caregiver time-off.

A quick search for caregiver- lists numerous resources, or sites that help track down resources and services. Caregiver.com caregiver.org caregiving.com etc... medicare has a link/resource for caregivers.

Caregiver Support Guide and Worksheet

Review: what are the annual additional medical expenses for caregivers? _____

What are some of the health-symptoms caregivers report?

_____

_____

_____

_____

Which of these symptoms do you also experience? Be honest. This is just for reference and starting points.   There is no judgment or recrimination.

_____

How often do I feel stressed, drained or depleted: Occasionally? Regularly? Often? Continually?

_____

What is your usual coping mechanism?

_____

_____

_____

_____

_____

Your stress is usually highest when:

_____

_____

_____

_____

List things that you do for yourself (healthy, or unhealthy):

1._____

2._____

3._____

4._____

Looking over the lists of foods, supplements and vitamins. A few that might be helpful for ME:

1._____

2._____

3._____

4._____

5._____

An activity or program I might try for myself:

1._____

2._____

Do I know someone who already engages in some activity, that I might like to try? What kinds of things do my friends/ social connections like to do?

_____

_____

_____

What are a few things I can do, at home, or on limited time, that might be rewarding or refreshing?

1._____

2._____

3._____

A grounding/ relaxation technique I might try is:

_____

The best time for me to be able to do this is:

_____

I might be interested in a social or online group that focuses on:

1._____

2._____

3._____

List one Mental, one physical and one emotional activity or component that you can try to incorporate regularly:

1._____

2._____

3._____

End Note

I hope you have found this information valuable, and that it improves the life and well-being of someone you know, love, or take care of. I invite you to take on a journey into a different approach to life. There are resources out there. New information is being discovered every day. The range of support available is vast. I intend to continue to develop this body of information, exploring modalities and protocols that can benefit the health and well-being of anyone who is cognitively challenged or struggles. Please also, visit my website for further resources and information. And share your stories and experiences there. I would love to hear both successes and failures. And your stories and information and experiences may help someone else along their way in this journey.

As noted and promised- here is my affiliate link for **Vitacost.com.** It is not any ONE single product that I am supporting here- but rather offering an excellent resource for finding reliable, trusted brands for holistic foods, vitamins, and supplements, with GREAT prices, and lots of special offers on a regular basis!

About Teri

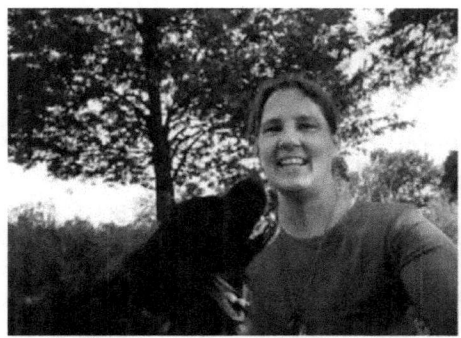 Teri brings her many years of work as a healer, herbalist and holistic coach to this project. Her background in education helps her to take important information and break it down into concepts that her students and readers can readily understand. She then finds ways to help them apply that learning into their lives, in ways that empowers them.

Teri has worked with her own health issues, through twenty years with chronic and non-responsive Lyme disease. This journey has taught her a lot about the immune system, the body's mechanism for detoxing, and cognitive and neurological functions and aspects.

She is a holistic coach, and specialises in at-risk youth, and chronic conditions. Her other works include Dancing in Your Bubble, a book that takes Andean Spirituality, and makes it comprehensible and practical for modern everyday life. She has also written "The power of animals: healing , intuition and grounding," as well as several shorter works and numerous blog-articles on her website: http://repairalz.com

She is a holistic coach, herbalist, bodyworker and author. She also works with rehab retired thoroughbred racehorses and teaches Holistic Equitation in Vermont, incorporating the concept of "building relationship," through working with horses.

Thank You for reading!

Dear Reader,

I hope you enjoyed the information in Holistic Support for Alzheimer's. This really came together for me as a labour of love, as much as a professional undertaking. I watched my mother recover from massive brain damage, as well as my own journey and struggle with cognitive-related issues (long term chronic Lyme disease which has neurological components that closely mirror the issues that Alzheimer's patients live with)... so I have personal and direct appreciation for the challenges the brain can encounter, PLUS its ability to return to optimal functioning- often against all odds and adverse conditions.

I also work as an herbalist, healer and holistic coach. In this work, I encounter a wide range of health issues. And I have worked particularly close with a couple of Alzheimer-dementia patients and their family/caregivers. It is a traumatic journey and experience- as you may well know, and appreciate.

I hope that you are able to benefit from the years of background, research and work that I have done, with supporting optimal health and brain health.

Also, please feel free to write me and let me know your thoughts and experiences. I will more than likely be working on a follow up at some point- so your information is valuable. Your input will help other people to benefit as well, from things you have learned and found on your own journeys through this experience. You can write HERE http://www.repairalz.com/contact/

Finally, I'd like to ask a favour. If you have a moment, I'd appreciate a review of the book. Love it, hate it, comments/ suggestions. You as the reader, in today's market, have the power to make or break a book. This is especially true with independent authors who are competing against the giant publishing houses. So if you have a minute, here is a link to my author page, on Amazon http://www.amazon.com/Teri-J.-Dluznieski-M.Ed./e/B003EN3DPY/ref=ntt_dp_epwbk_0

and you can sign up for updates on my site http://repairalz.com

Thank you so much for reading and for spending your valuable time with me.

Gratefully,

Teri J. Dluznieski M. Ed

If you liked this book, you may also be interested in
Dancing in Your Bubble (available at Amazon).

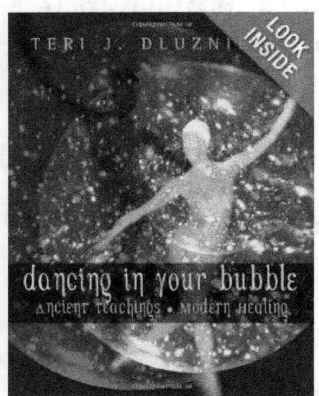

It is a book of practical Spiritual (non-denominational) teachings, based on the High Andes. But Mostly, it is the end result of my many years, teaching and healing. This book is the practical daily application of those years. How to understand and release stress, emotions and negative energy. How to live better, and stress-free in a very complicated and busy world.

Check out Teri's newest book: **Getting a Handle on Happy**: Improve Mental & Emotional health with Natural Healing Techniques and Nutrition   *Available March 2015 @ Amazon*

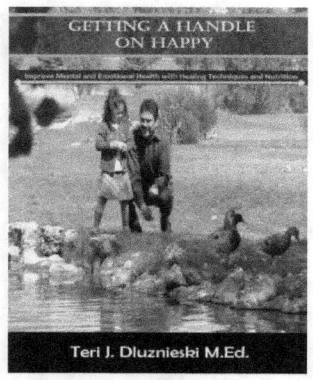